DR. CHARLES DAVID SPIVAK

TIMBERLINE BOOKS

Thomas J. Noel and Stephen J. Leonard, editors

The Beast, Benjamin Barr Lindsey with Harvey J. O'Higgins

Colorado's Japanese Americans, Bill Hosokawa

Denver: An Archaeological History, Sarah M. Nelson, K. Lynn Berry, Richard F. Carrillo, Bonnie L. Clark, Lori E. Rhodes, and Dean Saitta

Dr. Charles David Spivak: A Jewish Immigrant and the American Tuberculosis Movement, Jeanne E. Abrams

Ores to Metals: The Rocky Mountain Smelting Industry, James E. Fell, Jr.

A Tenderfoot in Colorado, R. B. Townshend

DR. CHARLES DAVID SPIVAK

A Jewish Immigrant and the American Tuberculosis Movement

Jeanne E. Abrams

UNIVERSITY PRESS OF COLORADO

Published by the University Press of Colorado
5589 Arapahoe Avenue, Suite 206C
Boulder, Colorado 80303

Printed in the United States of America

The University Press of Colorado is a proud member of
the Association of American University Presses.

The University Press of Colorado is a cooperative publishing enterprise supported, in part, by Adams State College, Colorado State University, Fort Lewis College, Mesa State College, Metropolitan State College of Denver, University of Colorado, University of Northern Colorado, and Western State College of Colorado.

The paper used in this publication meets the minimum requirements of the American National Standard for Information Sciences—Permanence of Paper for Printed Library Materials. ANSI Z39.48-1992

Library of Congress Cataloging-in-Publication Data

Abrams, Jeanne E., 1951–
Dr. Charles David Spivak : a Jewish immigrant and the American tuberculosis movement / Jeanne E. Abrams.
p. cm. — (Timberline books)
Includes bibliographical references and index.
ISBN 978-0-87081-941-4 (hardcover : alk. paper) 1. Spivak, C. D. (Charles D.), 1861–1927. 2. Jewish physicians—United States—Biography. 3. Jews, Russian—United States—Biography. 4. Jewish Consumptives' Relief Society (U.S.) 5. Tuberculosis—United States—History. I. Title.
R154.S68A27 2009
610.92—dc22
[B]

2009006558

Design by Daniel Pratt

18 17 16 15 14 13 12 11 10 09 10 9 8 7 6 5 4 3 2 1

Contents

Acknowledgments

When I interviewed Deena Spivak Strauss, the daughter of Dr. Charles David Spivak, in 1982 when I was working on my doctoral dissertation on the history of the Jewish Consumptives' Relief Society of Denver (JCRS), I had no premonition that more than twenty-five years later I would be completing a biography of her father. Yet even then I found Dr. Spivak's life extraordinarily fascinating as well as complex. I am very grateful for the many colleagues, friends, and family members who offered support, guidance, and valuable insights in the intervening years and helped bring this project to fruition. First, I extend a very special thank you to retired Philadelphia attorney and writer Harry Boonin, who first urged me to write a biography of Dr. Spivak so the doctor's remarkable life and career would become more well-known. Harry graciously shared his valuable and vivid primary sources on Spivak's early years in Philadelphia. I am grateful as well to Edward Ball, who generously made available his transcription of the diary of his grandfather, Dr.

Michael Ball. Dr. Ball was a close friend of Spivak's in Philadelphia in the late 1880s and early 1890s, and the diary proved to be an amazing resource. Dr. Spivak's family, including his late daughter Deena Spivak Strauss, and a number of his grandchildren—including Eugene and the late Dan Spivak, Adele Strauss Karsh, Ruth Strauss Oppenheim, the late Donald Strauss, and Charlesa Wolfe Feinstein—inherited their ancestor's highly engaging personality and were especially generous in sharing memories and photographs.

As always, I am indebted to numerous friends, colleagues, and "boosters" along the way. I am honored to be able to count Dr. Jonathan Sarna of Brandeis University and Dr. Alan Kraut of American University as esteemed colleagues as well as valued friends. Both carefully read drafts of the manuscript and, with their customary insight and wisdom, offered valuable suggestions. Darrin Pratt, director of the University Press of Colorado, offered encouragement from the beginning of the project, as did Dean Nancy Allen of Penrose Library and Provost Gregg Kvistad at the University of Denver. Thank you to my colleague Thyria Wilson for her expert assistance in preparing for publication the photographs that appear in this book. Dr. Stephen Leonard and Dr. Thomas Noel—the editors of the Timberline Series at the University Press of Colorado in which *Dr. Charles David Spivak: A Jewish Immigrant and the American Tuberculosis Movement* appears—added their valuable editorial skills, knowledge of Colorado history, and enthusiastic support. Finally, I have saved the best for last: my heartfelt appreciation to my loving family, including my husband, Lewis, and our children and grandchildren, for their unending support.

Foreword

Although more people probably came to Colorado for their physical health than for mineral wealth, the armies of "lungers" and "chasers" pursuing Colorado's renowned climate cure for tuberculosis, asthma, and other lung disorders never captured the attention that chambers of commerce and historians have lavished on gold and silver rushers. Yet these people spurred Colorado's growth and its emergence as a national leader in health care. Jeanne Abrams, a nationally recognized scholar and conservator of Western Jewish history, is a professor at Penrose Library at the University of Denver (DU). She also directs DU's Rocky Mountain Jewish Historical Society and Beck Archives, part of the Center for Judaic Studies and Penrose Library, and is the author of eight books and many articles, videos, and reviews.

Abrams's latest book is an important work of ethnic, medical, religious, and social history spotlighting a national notable unknown to the vast majority of Coloradans. Dr. Charles David Spivak published widely and worked with the leading warriors in fighting tuberculosis, the deadliest disease of his age. He also championed better health care for all and served as a leader for immigrants, advocating the preservation of ethnic and religious traditions in the more secular society of the United States. For his many patients, he was their "miracle man," who resourcefully provided whatever they needed, be it physical or spiritual. Yet the good doctor is little honored today.

A national leader in the crusade against tuberculosis, he was not only a scholar and researcher but also founded and led one of the nation's largest and most successful sanatoriums, Denver's Jewish Consumptives' Relief Society (JCRS), which served more than 10,000 patients for the fifty years after its 1904 founding.

In medical history, Spivak's work spans a key era of transition from religious- and ethnic-based volunteer charitable hospitals to modern, secular medical centers. During Spivak's 1861–1927 lifetime, the United States experienced its highest tides of immigrants, including more than 2 million Jews. One reaction to this influx was the rise of hate groups, such as the 1920s Ku Klux Klan, which targeted the Jewish immigrants Dr. Spivak served and defended. A Russian immigrant himself, Spivak respected newcomers' desires to hang on to their old country languages, cultures, and religion. Long before it was popular, he encouraged preserving these ethnic traditions, even if that meant slower Americanization.

Spivak's humanity is inspiring. Many tuberculosis sanatoriums did not want to deal with hopeless, dying patients, but Spivak contended that they were the ones most needing medical help. He saw patients not only as a body to cure but also as a soul to save. His compassionate and scientifically advanced treatment at the JCRS helped earn the high, dry, sunny state of Colorado its reputation as the "World's Sanatorium."

Thanks to Dr. Spivak's devotion to traditional Jewish *tzedakah* (charity, justice, and righteousness), JCRS was unusual in treating all patients at no charge and rarely imposing limits for stays. (Try requesting that next time you visit a doctor or hospital!) Furthermore, Spivak insisted that his staff "inaugurate a radical departure from similar institutions" by never treating patients as "public charges."

"Patients in a fragile emotional and physical state," as Abrams puts it, relished the personal attention from "Papa Spivak" and his staff, who wanted JCRS to be a home as well as a hospital. A visionary and idealistic socialist, Spivak brought to health care a far different approach than today's dollar-driven system of concentrating on those who can afford care.

While insisting that health care come from the heart, Spivak also used his head and experimented at JCRS with cutting-edge medical treatments, such as artificial pneumothorax surgery, which collapsed one lung to allow it to rest. Spivak wrote numerous medical articles in national journals and also became founding editor of *The Denver Jewish News*, forerunner of today's *Intermountain Jewish News.* He wrote for general as well as medical audiences, even penning Yiddish stories for leading Jewish periodicals in New York and Philadelphia.

Even in death, Spivak bridged the gap between traditional religion and modern science. His will requested a traditional Orthodox Jewish service but, contrary to Jewish law, gave his body to the Colorado Medical School for dissection. His articulated skeleton was shipped as a teaching aid to the Hebrew University in Jerusalem, but his viscera were buried, as he requested, in the Workman's Circle Section of the Jewish Golden Hill Cemetery on West Colfax Avenue, three miles west of the JCRS.

The JCRS closed in 1954 and the building was then used by the American Medical Center Cancer Research Center and later by the Rocky Mountain College of Art and Design. Today the largely preserved JCRS campus in the Denver suburb of Lakewood is on the National Register of Historic Places as a historic district. One original patient tent has been restored as an exhibit and the Isaac Solomon Synagogue is being restored for use as a museum.

Thanks to this newest addition to the University Press of Colorado's Timberline Series, Dr. Spivak has also been restored to prominence and his legacy as a physician, philanthropist, and Jewish "miracle man" documented.

THOMAS J. NOEL
CO-EDITOR, TIMBERLINE SERIES

DR. CHARLES DAVID SPIVAK

1

Introduction

"Anything my father needed for his patients . . . he got somehow. He was their miracle man, that's all I can say about my father." Although undoubtedly not an impartial observer, this is how Deena Spivak Strauss, the ninety-three-year-old daughter of Dr. Charles David Spivak,[1] recalled his life and work in a 1988 interview.[2] Charismatic, ambitious, highly intelligent, and articulate, but prone to pursue idealistic schemes, the reddish-blond-haired Spivak attracted followers wherever he went. In the first decades of the twentieth century he was a national leader in the crusade against tuberculosis as the executive secretary (director) of Denver's Jewish Consumptives' Relief Society (JCRS) sanatorium, one of the largest and best known of its kind in the United States. The JCRS opened in 1904 and served over 10,000 patients during its fifty-year existence as a tuberculosis sanatorium and hospital. Spivak was also a luminary in the American Jewish community, and his daughter's evaluation appears not to have been far off the mark. When he died in 1927, one of

Spivak's eulogizers characterized him as "one of the most popular figures in American medicine and in American Jewish life."[3] Physician, humanitarian, writer, linguist, journalist, administrator, social worker, ethnic broker, medical, public health, and social crusader—Dr. Charles Spivak was indeed a latter-day Renaissance man.

However, although Charles Spivak was certainly a fascinating, complex, and engaging figure, the story of his life rises above mere biography because it stands at the crossroads of so many critical junctures in American, western, Jewish, and medical history. Spivak's life and work serve as a wide lens through which to view myriad important topics, including the social construction of disease as related to ethnicity and class, the perceived connection specifically between immigrants and disease, and the transformation of the American hospital from a charitable, ethnic/religious–based voluntary institution to a modern corporate complex. They also reflect larger issues surrounding immigrant acculturation and intra-ethnic tensions, as well as how the concept of the Jew as an "outsider" at the turn of the twentieth century evolved into a phenomenon in which many of the outsiders became insiders who moved into the mainstream of American life. The story of Charles Spivak chronicles an immigrant's rise in America and the concurrent struggles between the Old World and the New World, reflecting the influence of class, religion, and regionalism. In addition, Spivak's career reflects pivotal emerging trends in public health, the culture of tuberculosis treatment, and changing medical thought about the nature of tuberculosis itself—encompassing the debate over whether tuberculosis was a physiological or a social-based disease, the best manner in which to deal with epidemics, and tensions between religion and science.

Between Spivak's birth in 1861 and his death in 1927, the United States experienced massive immigration, rapid industrialization, and increased urbanization. Some of the transformations on the American landscape were reflected in Progressive-Era ideology that influenced innovations in medical treatment and public health philosophy and the increased professionalization of health and medicine. The great tide of immigration between 1880 and 1925, with its significant Jewish component of well over 2 million, was particularly critical within the American Jewish community. During the peak years of immigration, from about 1900 to 1910, only Italians outnumbered East European Jewish arrivals; Jewish immigrants, driven out of their homelands by discrimination, persecution, and poverty, made America their permanent home.[4] That near tidal wave of immigration became a major factor in the changing of the guard in the leadership of American Jewry from the older, established, and acculturated Jews—who had emigrated largely from German states—to the East European newcomers. In 1880 only one out of every six American Jews was of East European origin; by 1920, five out of six American Jews hailed from East Europe.

The peak of Jewish immigration intersected with the rise of the American tuberculosis movement and the proliferation of tuberculosis sanatoriums throughout the United States, especially in the West. Although East European Jewish immigrants actually demonstrated a lower incidence of tuberculosis compared to other religious and ethnic groups, anti-immigrant and anti-Semitic stereotypes often appeared that accused Jews of being carriers of a number of diseases, and tuberculosis was often referred to pejoratively as the "Jewish disease."[5] The association of disease and germs with immigrants and the poor only exacerbated underlying feelings of nativism and prejudice that surfaced as the nation saw a significant increase in general immigration during the last decades of the nineteenth century and the beginning of the twentieth century.[6] It is no accident that the American Jewish community played a leading role in the founding of tuberculosis sanatoriums or hospitals around the country, most of them at least formally nonsectarian. The opening of Jewish tuberculosis treatment centers had at least two underlying motivations: to demonstrate commitment to treating the disease as a reflection of the broader Jewish civic sense of responsibility and to dispel prevalent negative notions about Jewish immigrants.

No single accepted standard for tuberculosis treatment prevailed in America in the early years, but by the 1880s medical opinion had begun to emphasize fresh air, rest, diet, climate, and a controlled environment in the treatment of the disease. Physicians and public health officials increasingly viewed the sanatorium as the best place to aid victims and to isolate them from the general population as germ theory developed and fear of contagion spread. In a prize-winning booklet published in 1901, Dr. Adolphus Knopf lauded the curative benefits of the sanatorium lifestyle and maintained that in such a "modern" institution characterized by "hygienic and preventive measures . . . one is in less danger of becoming infected with the germs of consumption there than anywhere else."[7] In

1900 there were only 34 sanatoriums in the United States, but by 1925 the number had climbed to over 500, reflecting the growing popularity of the institution nationally.[8]

Despite Robert Koch's discovery of the tubercle bacillus in 1882, through the late nineteenth and early twentieth centuries most physicians continued to view tuberculosis as caused by a combination of bacterial infection *and* specific social conditions.[9] Tuberculosis therefore was unique as a disease, as during the modern era health crusaders increasingly perceived it as an illness with specific roots in congested urban environments, characterized by crowded and unsanitary working and living conditions, and as on one level a "social disease rooted in poverty and poor housing."[10] Thus, the social as well as biological underpinnings of the disease were frequently emphasized, and sanatoriums like Denver's JCRS exhibited both a medical and a social component. In this context, the sanatorium served as an educational tool to alter "unhealthy" lifestyles and encourage good habits, as a means of removing the poor from crowded urban areas, and as a medical environment for treating infection through rest, nutritious foods, fresh air, sunlight, and at times surgical intervention.

While some upscale sanatoriums such as Cragmor in Colorado Springs served the upper and upper middle classes, most of them treated the genteel poor, the working classes, and the destitute.[11] Additionally, many physicians prescribed a "certain climate" as part of tuberculosis treatment. The American West and Colorado in particular, with its dry, sunny environment and high altitude, fit the "prescription" perfectly. In short order the state became known as the "World's Sanatorium."[12] Historians are increasingly beginning to recognize the connection between environmental and medical history and the perceived therapeutic landscape of region.[13] Certain areas were seen as more efficacious for tuberculosis victims than others, and, as one author has observed in regard to consumptives, "for most Americans salvation lay not to the south but to the west."[14]

By the time of Spivak's death in 1927, many health care institutions initially begun as ethnic hospitals to serve immigrants had evolved into something altogether different, with a progressive weakening of the hospitals' relationship to the ethnic communities from which they had originated.[15] At the turn of the twentieth century, however, the ethnic component of the majority of health care institutions—the JCRS among them—was still of major importance, as "an ethnic or religious community's honor was in some sense at stake in providing for its own."[16] Moreover, "ethnic and religious groups saw their [medical] institutions as symbols of community identity and responsibility."[17] The JCRS had much in common with other sanatoriums around the country from a purely medical treatment standpoint. However, as a result of pervasive East European Jewish cultural, social, and religious influences, as well as western regional currents, it often differed in outlook and philosophy from other religious- and ethnic-based institutions. Animated by traditional Jewish concepts of *tzedakah* (commonly translated as charity but literally meaning "justice" or "righteousness"), the JCRS's emphasis on treating all patients at no charge, as well as accepting patients in all stages of the disease and rarely imposing limits for stays, contrasted markedly with common policy at most sanatorium/hospitals. In addition, according to Dr. Philip Hillkowitz, the first president of the JCRS, the institution also incorporated a "breezy western species" of democracy into its operation.[18]

Although tuberculosis in the nineteenth century was certainly no respecter of class or ethnic group, by the turn of the century it was evident that the poor—especially immigrants—suffered disproportionately from the disease.[19] Many in the Jewish community came to believe that treating Jewish patients, especially consumptives, in a welcoming environment that respected their cultural practices and religious beliefs contributed to an improvement in their health. This was one central factor in the founding of over sixty Jewish hospitals or sanatoriums in the United States between 1850 and 1930.[20] In this context, Dr. Charles Spivak played a key role in the lives of Jewish immigrant patients from throughout the United States as an immigrant cultural "broker" or mediator in his central position at the JCRS. This was accomplished by simultaneously easing these immigrants into American society, introducing them to American culture, and nurturing their ethnic traditions at the same time—a role more commonly associated with politicians, journalists, and the clergy. Historian Alan Kraut has noted that immigrant physicians who belonged to a variety of ethnic groups around the country were becoming sensitive to the fact that in treating fellow immigrant newcomers, "the balance between assimilation and cultural integrity was at stake."[21]

Paradoxically but not surprisingly considering his strong Jewish and socialist ties, while Spivak considered himself a "modern" and "scientific" man, he rejected the Progressive-Era business model for hospitals and other charitable institutions. In an early editorial written for the JCRS publication *The Sanatorium*, Spivak railed against what he termed the contemporary so-called scientific and sociological methods for dispensing aid. He claimed that personal and human elements were entirely lacking in such an approach and urged instead that charity be "of the heart, and not of the head."[22]

While some historians have characterized early sanatoriums, particularly the larger ones, as "prison-like,"[23] this was not the case at the JCRS. Despite firm rules and regulations and a somewhat paternalistic tone at the sanatorium, the JCRS exhibited a family-like ambiance, largely because of the influence of Spivak and his close friend and longtime president of the JCRS, Dr. Philip Hillkowitz, the son of a leading Denver East European Orthodox Jewish rabbi. One early observer maintained that JCRS patients were fortunate to be "in an institution where they are treated as brothers and where they may maintain their self-respect and at the same time regain their health."[24] A woman who had been a patient at both the Denver National Jewish Hospital for Consumptives (NJH) (founded by a group of largely acculturated German Jews) and, later, the JCRS in the 1920s commented that "NJH was a hospital, but the JCRS was a home."[25]

Moreover, Spivak had great disdain for popular contemporary philanthropy that dispensed charity in an often condescending, patronizing, moralistic manner and only to those considered "worthy" recipients. Spivak insisted that charity patients be treated with dignity and respect. In 1905, in his first report as secretary, Spivak maintained that the JCRS intended to "inaugurate a radical departure from similar organizations, by eliminating from the conduct and management of the Sanatorium, anything and everything that would tend to remind the inmates of the fact that they are 'public charges.'"[26] This statement reflected Spivak's outlook on life, a rather unique blend of Yiddishkeit, socialism, and secularism. While Spivak was foremost a physician and tuberculosis crusader, as two prominent medical historians have observed, "[m]edical history can inform us as much about general social and political change as about science and medicine."[27] Spivak's life allows us a firsthand view into all these areas.

While the interactive style exhibited by many physicians and their patients in hospital/sanatorium settings in the late nineteenth and early twentieth centuries often appears highly paternalistic to our contemporary sensibilities, at the time, many patients in a fragile emotional and physical state welcomed the personal attention. Spivak was closely involved in the lives of his patients at the JCRS in a manner that extended far beyond mere medical treatment. He was affectionately called "Papa Spivak" by those he treated, and they often turned to him for advice and guidance. He was not reluctant to voice his opinions and offer his personal code of morality. A letter Dr. Spivak wrote in 1907 to a former patient who had returned to Des Moines, Iowa, reflects, in a humorous yet revealing manner, the close relationships he forged with patients. Spivak had been asked for advice concerning the possibility of the man marrying a young woman he had recently met. The good doctor replied that he felt the young man's tuberculosis condition had improved, but not to the point that he should marry: "Marriage will retard your recovery. . . . You say that the girl is not good looking, but she has money. I don't think it is right to marry [for] money. You did not say a word whether you like the girl or not. If she likes you and you like her, then she can wait a year or two until you recover your health completely."[28]

Always genial, optimistic, and energetic, his innate personality, upbringing, and historical roots also made Dr. Charles David Spivak a man of intense contradictions. Born in 1861 into a traditionally observant Russian Jewish family, like many of his contemporaries he became attracted to Haskala, or Jewish Enlightenment, currents as a student. He became a revolutionary socialist in his youth and was forced to flee Russia in 1882 to escape being apprehended by the Russian secret police for his radical political activities. Spivak arrived first in New York City, where he began work as a typesetter for *The Jewish Messenger* and renewed acquaintances with other Russian-born Jewish socialists. He subsequently labored for a time as a road paver on New York's Fifth Avenue and as a mill hand in Maine before receiving a medical degree with honors from Jefferson Medical College in Philadelphia in 1890.[29]

Although sometimes criticized for being a dreamer, Spivak's potential seemed evident from the beginning. When he received a first prize gold medal at his graduation for a winning essay on obstetrics, *The Jewish Messenger* lauded him as "one of the most intelligent young men who immigrated to this country from Russia in the tide of 1882."[30] A professed freethinker, Spivak also delighted in a traditional Jewish ceremony in Philadelphia in 1893 when he wed fellow Russian immigrant Jennie Charsky, a kindred spirit with radical anarchist leanings. He also followed tradition with a customary Jewish *bris,* or circumcision ceremony, for the couple's son David, born that same year.[31]

As a result of Jennie's ill health, in 1896 the Spivaks moved to Denver, a magnet for tuberculosis victims. Charles soon opened a private practice and later became a founder and the "guiding genius" of the JCRS, which became one of America's leading tuberculosis sanatoriums. In addition to his medical responsibilities, Spivak supervised fundraising operations at the JCRS and chronicled the history, activities, and patient statistics at the institution as a regular contributor and later editor of its bimonthly official publication, *The Sanatorium*. He also became a leading figure in Colorado's medical community, teaching on the faculty of Denver's School of Medicine as a lecturer on gastrointestinal diseases—his specialty—and later as a professor of anatomy and clinical medicine, serving on the boards of several medical societies, and volunteering as the librarian of the Denver Academy of Medicine.

In 1899 the National Jewish Hospital for Consumptives had opened in Denver, largely supported by affluent Jews primarily of German descent.[32] The JCRS was founded in 1904 by a number of Russian Jewish immigrants, including Spivak, who felt the NJH sometimes treated its largely destitute patients in a condescending manner and was frequently insensitive to the religious traditions of many East European immigrant Jews. At the helm of the JCRS, Charles Spivak was able to merge his fierce commitment to medicine and science with his socialist and Jewish roots. His intense concern for humanity in general and Jewish imperatives of charity in particular prompted him to insist that the JCRS accept patients in all stages of the disease free of charge, a radical departure from conventional medical wisdom at the time. Progressive-Era philosophy, concerned as it was with efficiency and rationality, generally dictated that only those patients with incipient tuberculosis who had the best chance for a cure should be treated. Under Spivak's guidance, the JCRS was also a cutting-edge pioneer in the introduction of artificial pneumothorax surgical intervention, in which one lung was collapsed in an attempt to allow it to rest. Although the procedure sometimes proved dangerous and was ultimately of dubious long-term medical benefit, contemporary medical thought found it promising, and it became a popular form of treatment.[33] Between 1911 and the late 1940s, thousands of pneumothorax procedures were performed at the JCRS, with nearly 1,400 in 1948 alone.[34]

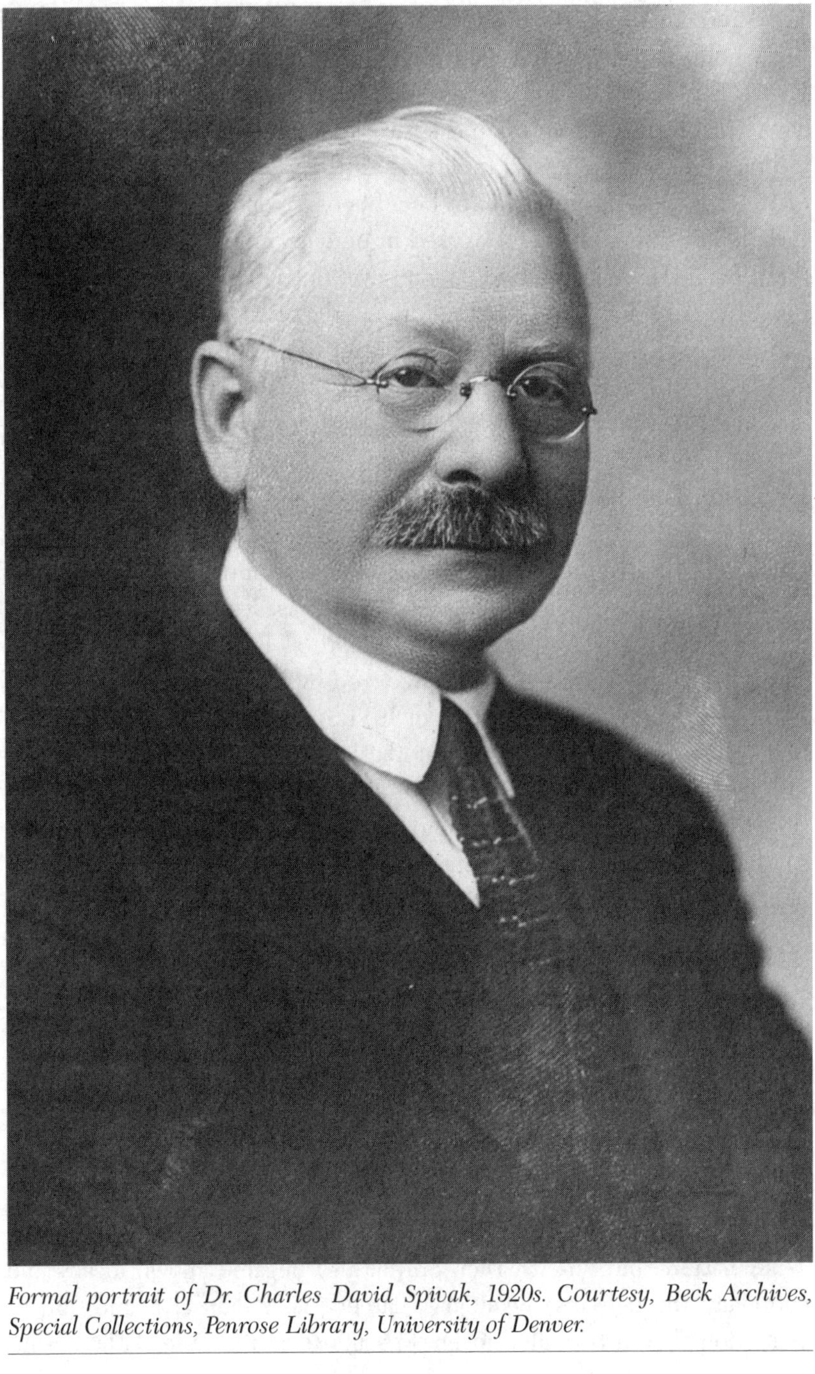

Formal portrait of Dr. Charles David Spivak, 1920s. Courtesy, Beck Archives, Special Collections, Penrose Library, University of Denver.

Although the JCRS sanatorium was formally nonsectarian, most of the patients and many of the consulting physicians through the 1930s were Jewish. Spivak and his colleagues also fostered a visible Jewish atmosphere at the institution, which offered kosher food and Yiddish discourse and exhibited respect for Jewish traditions. At the same time, Spivak and other JCRS leaders appreciated the benefits of America for themselves and their fellow immigrants and worked in perhaps a more sensitive manner than the NJH to acculturate patients without ignoring Jewish sensibilities. Therefore, for example, American holidays such as the Fourth of July and Thanksgiving were celebrated with great enthusiasm (as they were at NJH), but the festivities included kosher refreshments and emphasis on the compatibility of American and Jewish ideals. In fact, Spivak's own eclectic philosophy strongly influenced JCRS policies, reflecting no doubt his personal odysseys from alien to American and from secularist to committed Jew.

The JCRS was probably the first and most significant national Jewish institution founded, funded, and guided by East European Jews, and on one level the JCRS was perhaps an attempt to "democratize" Jewish philanthropy in the United States. Influenced by his socialist beliefs, at the JCRS's tenth anniversary meeting in 1914 Spivak proudly reported: "The first lesson [the JCRS] taught was that a national organization can be brought into the world without the midwifery of the rich and the professional philanthropist. . . . It proved to the world that a national organization can be launched, built and maintained by small tradesmen and workingmen, the so called hoi-polloi."[35]

Spivak insisted that the JCRS be a "peoples' institution," with money collected from thousands of working-class supporters with modest incomes from throughout the country, a policy that diverged from the norm but that proved successful from an economic standpoint for decades. In 1906 Spivak advised Anna Hillkowitz, one of the JCRS's traveling field workers/fundraisers, "I think you should abandon entirely the idea of making any strenuous effort to meet our rich brethren. If our Institution is to be a peoples' institution, it should be supported by the people only. Let us collect our moneys in dollars and quarters."[36]

A natural and gifted writer, Spivak also became known locally and nationally through his secondary "career" as a journalist and author. "Attention should be called to Dr. Spivak's scientific style. Although his work is accurate and couched in scientific terms, his scientific papers read easily. There is a certain flavor to his philosophic and literary interjections that make [sic] his writings most interesting."[37] That is how fellow physician Dr. A. Levinson described Dr. Charles Spivak's engaging writing style. It reveals both Spivak's easy facility with the English language—all the more remarkable because of his immigrant origins—and his medical expertise as a physician and man of science, as well as his lifelong love affair with the written word through books, periodicals, and newspapers. His daughter, Deena Spivak Strauss, recalled that her father always carried a pencil and paper in his pocket so he could jot down a new idea or concept that came to him as he made his rounds and fulfilled the demands of his busy schedule.[38] Indeed, his personal file box at the JCRS is filled with handwritten notes and outlines on a variety of subjects, including medical and Jewish topics, which probably served as the basis of many of his articles and speeches.[39]

In addition to publishing medical articles in prominent journals, he became the founding editor of *The Denver Jewish News*, forerunner of *The Intermountain Jewish News*. In 1911 he coauthored a nationally recognized popular Yiddish dictionary with well-known Yiddish poet Yehoash (Solomon Bloomgarden), a patient at the JCRS for a time. For several years in the 1920s Spivak penned a series of popular articles in Yiddish for the Jewish daily *The Forward* on topics concerning health and hygiene with such intriguing titles as "Counsel of Wise People on Long Life" and "Don't Crawl into a Clean Bed with Dirty Feet."[40] Together with his friend and fellow Russian immigrant Abraham Cahan, the famous editor of *The Forward*, Spivak utilized the newspaper as a vehicle for acculturating Yiddish-speaking Jewish immigrants into American norms and imparting public health directives in a nonthreatening manner. In 1920, nearing age sixty, Charles Spivak undertook a harrowing trip to Poland as special commissioner of the American Jewish Joint Distribution Committee (JDC) to aid World War I victims and study the health conditions of European Jews. Spivak's appointment to the position reflected both the respect he commanded within the American Jewish community and his commitment to social work among his co-religionists.

"Papa Spivak," as he was known at the JCRS, eventually achieved middle-class respectability and a national reputation, but to the end he remained faithful to his East European co-religionists and his early socialist principles. An individualist from his youth, Charles Spivak was recalled as having a "many-sided" personality by close friend Isaac Rivkind, a librarian at New York's Jewish Theological Seminary. Rivkind related that on a short visit to New York in April 1927, within only twenty-four hours Spivak managed to attend a meeting of Hebrew-speaking physicians; a banquet hosted by *Hadoar*, a Hebrew periodical; and a meeting of Jewish communists discussing plans to celebrate May Day, and he also participated in the cornerstone celebration of the Orthodox Jewish Rabbi Isaac Elchanan Seminary.[41]

Even at Spivak's death his contradictory spirit lingered on. In his will he instructed that his funeral be conducted in accordance with Orthodox Jewish customs, but at the same time he requested that his body be dissected (in most cases a violation of traditional Jewish law) and the bones and organs shipped to the University of Jerusalem to be utilized for training future physicians in anatomy classes in the interest of science. His remaining viscera were then buried at Denver's Golden Hill Cemetery in the section reserved for many of his beloved patients.[42]

In 1889 Dr. Michael Ball, a friend and colleague of the young Spivak, then a struggling and impoverished medical student in Philadelphia, observed in his diary: "I hope to see him [Spivak] someday famous, he deserves it."[43] Ball's words proved prescient. In 1915 Spivak returned to Philadelphia to deliver a well-attended public lecture on tuberculosis. Along with Spivak the presenters included Dr. Solomon Solis-Cohen, a noted Philadelphia doctor, and Dr. Lawrence Flick, renowned American tuberculosis crusader, director of Pennsylvania's first successful sanatorium, and founder of the first voluntary tuberculosis organization in America—the Pennsylvania Society for the Prevention of Tuberculosis. A University of Pennsylvania physician introduced the three physicians as the "super-dreadnoughts of their profession."[44]

When Charles Spivak died in 1927, letters and telegrams of condolence poured in from all corners of the United States, and his obituary appeared in newspapers around the country. In one published eulogy, his longtime friend and colleague, Denver's Dr. Philip Hillkowitz, commented on Spivak's ideological roots: "A product of the Russian liberal movement of the eighties, Dr. Spivak had imbibed in his formative period the idealism of that urge to go to the people."[45] That compulsion to be of service to his fellow Jews and humankind as a whole would shape Spivak's career and lifestyle until his untimely death from cancer at age sixty-five. Leading American Jewish educator and social worker Dr. Boris Bogen, who had accompanied Spivak to Poland as the general director of JDC European relief operations, characterized his close friend and fellow immigrant as a "scientist, a scholar and an idealist. He was a thinker and a dreamer at the same time. As a social worker he was unconventional."[46]

However, the story of the life of Dr. Charles David Spivak is much more than the biography of an individual physician—albeit a remarkable one—for it stands at the crossroads of American, Jewish, medical, and immigration history and broadens our understanding of the history of public health in America. Moreover, it highlights the key role Colorado played in the treatment of tuberculosis as well as the roles particular physicians played in the state's development. It also illuminates how the widespread threat of tuberculosis, the leading cause of death in the United States at the turn of the twentieth century, transformed the American landscape through social and cultural influences that extended far beyond the field of medicine. As social historian Sheila Rothman has noted, the disease not only helped shape public policy but also affected personal habits, including "everything from the length of women's skirts to the design of tenement houses."[47] Indeed, tuberculosis became a "national preoccupation" and the source of a miniature economy,[48] perhaps nowhere more visibly than in Colorado.

The efficacy of the sanatorium continues to be debated to this day—the sanatorium offered treatment rather than a cure, and the mortality rate at the JCRS and other sanatoriums around the country that accepted patients with advanced cases of tuberculosis remained discouragingly high.[49] For example, despite years at the well-known Saranac Lake tuberculosis treatment center, which he directed, Dr. Edward Trudeau—the "father" of the American sanatorium movement—continued during most of his adult life to suffer from the disease, which eventually claimed his life. Moreover, by the 1880s the tuberculosis rate had already been exhibiting a decline that predated the proliferation of sanatoriums. However, the sanatorium phenomenon played a leading role on the American scene for many decades. Regardless of how we view the tuberculosis movement in retrospect, as historian and physician Barbara Bates has pointed out, at the time "[p]hysicians, nurses, politicians, social leaders, officials of tuberculosis societies, and doubtless much of the public all believed that the tuberculosis movement was scientific, socially justifiable, and somehow effective."[50] Certainly, isolating tuberculosis patients from the general population helped stem the spread of the disease. Ultimately, the JCRS sanatorium under the direction of Dr. Spivak served the American Jewish community by providing a supportive haven in which to "chase the cure" that facilitated tuberculosis treatment as well as the transition of Jewish immigrant patients into Jewish American citizens.

The discovery of a host of new drugs—including streptomycin and later isoniazid—as well as generally improving socioeconomic conditions and wider public health reforms were among the most important factors that helped bring tuberculosis under control, although the disease was never eradicated as hoped.[51] However, effective chemotherapy signaled the demise of the sanatorium. In 1954 Trudeau's famed Saranac Lake sanatorium closed, the same year the JCRS transferred its mission to cancer research and treatment and became the American Medical Center.

In a recent speech before the Immigration and Ethnic History Society, leading medical and immigration historian Alan Kraut urged other historians to acknowledge "the role that health and disease play in shaping patterns of international migration and cultural integration."[52] Spivak's life story, compelling as it is, opens a window on American life in the first decades of the twentieth century and gains even greater significance in what it reveals about wider national issues such as health care, ethnicity, immigration, acculturation, and moral and ethical questions concerning responsibility for the sick and indigent—questions that continue to command our attention to this day. Perhaps most important, Dr. Charles David Spivak epitomized the physician who understood and shaped health policy in a way that was sensitive to the connection between culture and medicine at a time when few others appreciated the link.

2

Out of Russia

Turbulent Tsarist Russia, home to the largest number of Jews in Europe in the late nineteenth century,[1] provided a heady atmosphere for reformers and revolutionaries. As Orthodox Jewish customs and institutions came under assault by liberal Haskala, or Jewish Enlightenment, ideology filtering in from Western Europe and Russian officials offered limited opportunities to Jews to promote selective integration into Russian society, some young Jewish men and women distanced themselves from traditional Jewish life. Many whose native tongue was Yiddish learned the Russian language, became admirers of Russian literature and culture, and were drawn to competing political movements such as socialism, nihilism, populism, and even anarchism. As Steven Cassedy put it succinctly in *To the Other Shore*, his study of Russian Jewish intellectuals, they became "Russified, secularized, then politicized."[2]

This was the pattern followed by Charles David Spivak, who was born Chaim Dovid Spivakofsky in Kremenchug, in the state of Poltava in southern Russia, on December 25, 1861. Kremenchug was located on the Dnieper River in Russian Poland, part of the notorious "Pale of Settlement," where the majority of Russian Jews lived as a result of Tsarist legal restrictions governing Jewish residence. It was established around 1570, and Jewish life in the town dated back to the late eighteenth century. In 1897 the Jewish population there was close to 30,000, nearly half of the city's total number. Kremenchug became a commercial center of note and at times boasted a substantial Jewish populace, which was considerably reduced during World War II following occupation by the Nazis. Jews in Kremenchug generally made a living in traditional occupations as tailors, small shopkeepers, peddlers, or brokers.

Relatively few Jews at the time Spivak was growing up were allowed to settle in the Russian interior, the site of most of Russia's major cities, including Moscow and St. Petersburg. Spivak was the son of Orthodox Jewish parents, Samuel David and Deborah Adel Dorfman Spivakofsky. Samuel was fifteen years older than his wife, and Chaim was the only surviving son of the eleven children Deborah had borne. The young Spivak received a traditional Jewish education in Kremenchug, studying with his father as well as attending a *cheder* (a Jewish religious elementary school). Chaim also received a strong grounding in the study of higher-level Talmudic texts. In addition to his Jewish studies, Spivak, who was gifted at languages, became fluent in Russian. Always a voracious reader, Spivak secretly read secular newspapers and whatever popular and classical literature he could get his hands on, and he was undoubtedly familiar with the anti-czarist and Haskala literature of the day. He became sufficiently self-educated in secular subjects to pass the examination to enter the local secondary-level Russian gymnasium. Disenchanted with general social conditions, legal disabilities imposed on Jews, and the repressive, authoritarian Russian government, he became a member of the radical left and joined the Socialist Revolutionary Party while studying for university admittance.[3]

In his aspirations for higher education, Spivak was only one of many young Jews who took advantage of more open nineteenth-century Russian education admission policies, although there were quotas in place. Jews in Russia had long suffered officially sanctioned legal, economic, social, and religious restrictions, which included constraints on one's choice of career, place of residence, and ability to own property and which continued

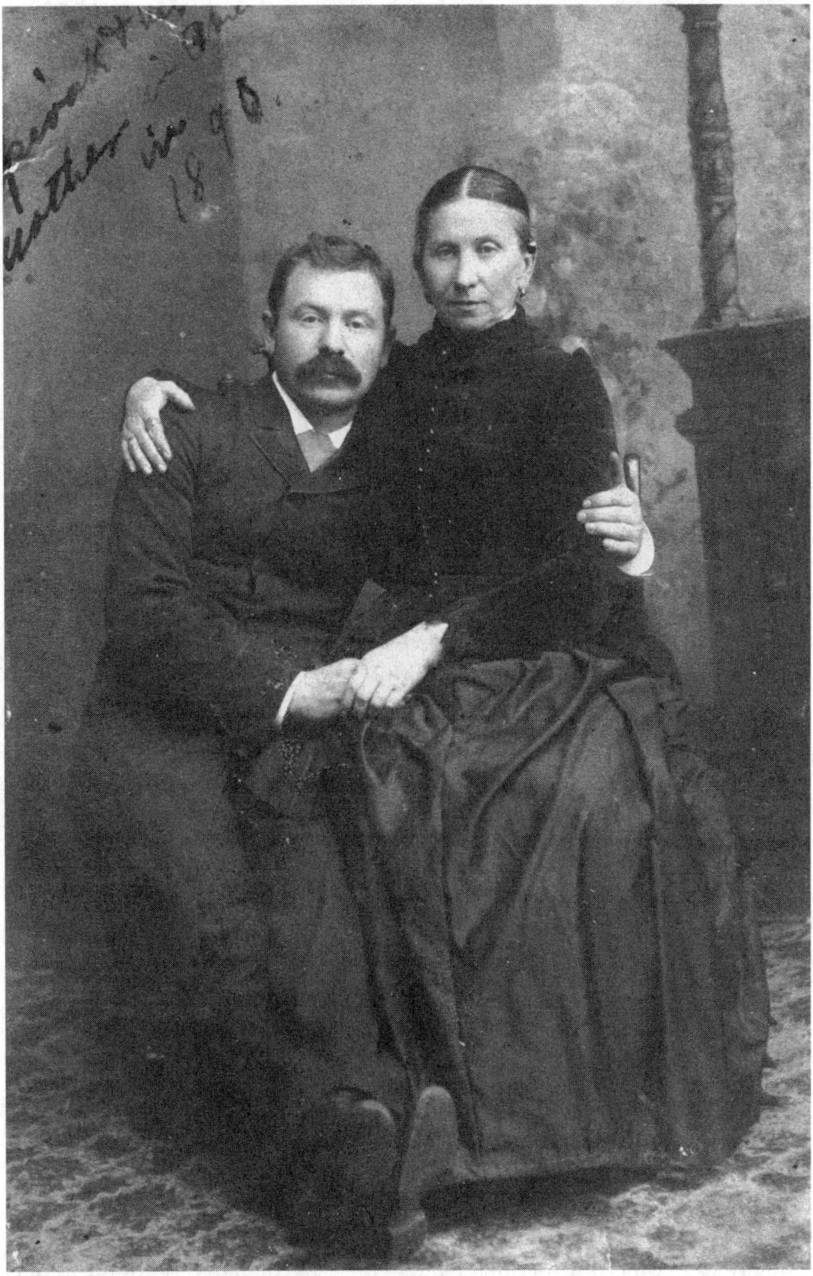

Portrait of Dr. Charles David Spivak with his mother, Deborah, in Philadelphia, 1890. Courtesy, Charlesa Wolfe Feinstein.

through the nineteenth and early twentieth centuries. However, beginning in the early nineteenth century, in a pragmatic effort to integrate the Jewish population into general Russian society, official government policy allowed Jewish boys and girls to enter state-sponsored secular schools and by 1880 allowed about 60,000 Jews to reside outside the Pale. Once Jews were legally allowed to enter higher-level Russian secular schools, they flocked to these gymnasiums and universities in disproportionate numbers. As part of a selective Russian integration policy specifically directed toward Jews, between 1861 and 1887 young Jews were encouraged to enter state-run secular educational institutions, and they formed "the seed bed of a Russian-Jewish intelligentsia."[4] Moreover, historian Benjamin Nathans has argued provocatively that not only was the Russian Empire a place from which Jews fled, but it also provided them with an incubator for political and social reform and innovation—particularly in the case of institutions of higher learning, which nurtured the revolutionary movement.[5]

Indeed, Spivak later recalled that liberal political ideas imported from America formed an important part of both his and his fellow Jewish radicals' ideological development while they still lived in Russia. Among the "revolutionary" texts the young activists devoured were Russian translations of the Declaration of Independence and the U.S. Constitution alongside Russian writings on radical philosophies. Certainly, Spivak was exposed early on to a wide and eclectic range of political thought.[6]

Only a small percentage of Jews in the Russian Empire were actually familiar with socialist ideas before coming to America or participated in revolutionary organizations there in the 1870s and 1880s.[7] Charles Spivak was among that small group of young Jews who had adopted a socialist ideology *before* arriving in the United States. One contemporary recalled that Spivak was inspired to join a revolutionary circle at age sixteen after reading *Ha-Emet* (The Truth), a radical Hebrew Russian newspaper published by Jewish revolutionaries.[8] According to his boyhood Russian friend Victor Yarros (Yaroslavsky), Spivak was an individualist even as a teenager. Yarros met Spivak when they were aspiring university students in Kremenschug and were preoccupied with preparing for entrance exams. Yet they occasionally took time out for social gatherings, particularly to attend underground meetings of the local branch of the Socialist Revolutionary Party, whose lofty mission was to transform the inequitable social order of the

Russian Empire. Like many members of the idealistic Jewish intelligentsia, Spivak and Yarros shared a common ideological background and passionately discussed the burning issues of the day at these get-togethers. Spivak's future avocation as a writer was also presaged during this period, as he worked on the group's revolutionary newsletter and contributed a "light and satirical" article that mocked the Russian authorities. Spivak's writing talent emerged at an early age. Yarros observed that his friend "had a gift for humor and irony, and wrote well to boot."[9]

Participation in radical political activities and the pursuit of idealistic goals rather than specific religious persecution, social discrimination, or economic deprivation were the primary factors that precipitated Spivak's emigration to America. The Russian Jewish intellectuals of the period identified with the general Russian intelligentsia and often admired and adopted their revolutionary, utopian ideology and radical thought. Many Jewish intellectuals had thus been "convinced that the only life worth living was a life of service."[10] Undoubtedly, Chaim Spivak's early desire to "live a life of service," prompted by socialist principles, foreshadowed his later decision to go into medicine, particularly his inclination to first assist impoverished Jewish immigrants and later to concentrate on those doubly afflicted with tuberculosis and poverty.

Yarros provides a dramatic account, perhaps heightened by the distance of time, of his and Spivak's flight from their homeland. With other members of his revolutionary band, Spivak had distributed forbidden radical newspapers and books smuggled in from Moscow, and before long the Russian secret police acted to eliminate the perceived threat. A crackdown on radicals, particularly Jewish ones, ensued following the assassination of Czar Alexander II in 1881. The nascent reform movement suffered a great setback with Alexander's death, and the police reacted to the assassination by curtailing civil liberties. Even though only one Jew was involved in the assassination conspiracy, it triggered bloody anti-Jewish pogroms. Spivak was living with an aunt in Kremenchug at the time, and he and Yarros were betrayed by one of their cohorts. When his aunt's house was surrounded, Spivak escaped arrest because "his clever aunt, who knew everything, had contrived to throw the revolutionary pamphlets and papers into a cabbage barrel."[11]

Both Spivak and Yarros were detained by the police and after a grueling interrogation were dismissed with a severe warning. They were clearly in danger. Many of their comrades had been imprisoned and some executed to serve as an example to other aspiring revolutionaries. The leaders of the local Socialist Revolutionary Party financed a theatrical escape for Spivak and Yarros. In the early morning hours they were secretly put on a train to Kiev. As young Jewish men over sixteen and thus of potential military age were not allowed to leave Russia, they lacked necessary legal emigration papers. Spivak and Yarros were subsequently smuggled across the Russian-Austrian border and celebrated their escape in an Austrian inn.[12] Through word of mouth the United States had gained a wide reputation as a "golden land" among Russian Jews and other immigrant groups throughout Europe, and Spivak and Yarros were attracted to the dream shared by many oppressed immigrants. As a contemporary of Spivak's put it, "Rays of hope came to us from a far distant land—the United States of America."[13] According to Yarros, "America, the land of the free and of opportunity, was our ultimate destination," and in short order he and Spivak boarded a ship sailing from the port of Hamburg, Germany, and arrived in New York City in May 1882.[14]

Undoubtedly, Spivak initially passed through Castle Garden, the New York State Emigration Depot, located at the tip of Manhattan. Castle Garden began operations in 1855. In 1891 the federal government took over the immigration process, and Ellis Island, America's major immigration center, opened in 1892. Spivak's arrival in New York City coincided with the surge in Russian Jewish immigration following the repression sparked by the czar's murder. By 1880 about a third of American Jews lived in New York, and thousands of the early Russian Jewish immigrants settled in the tenement area of the city's Lower East Side. By 1910 more than 500,000 Jews were crammed into a one-and-a-half-square-mile area.[15] Shortly after his arrival, Spivak probably adopted the English name Charles to reflect his American persona, but his Jewish immigrant friends continued to call him Chaim.

Yarros reported that he and Spivak had hoped to join a "progressive" agricultural settlement (a quasi-commune in Oregon composed of Russian immigrants) and "become tillers of the soil, applying, however, our radical ideas—ideas of co-operation, fraternity, altruism, service." The idealistic colony unraveled before the two could migrate, however, and like so many other Russian immigrants, Spivak was forced to find menial work on the East Coast.[16] Indeed, this was the fate of most of those who participated in similar utopian experiments, especially those founded by Jewish immigrants, which failed around the country.

Despite the common radical revolutionary and socialist alliances and what Joseph Brandes has identified as a secular rather than religious-based "universal humanism" prevalent among his socialist contemporaries, Spivak, an individualist, from his earliest years also closely aligned himself with the Jewish community.[17] Most Jewish revolutionists were alienated from the Jewish people, whom they felt clung to backward customs. Instead, the revolutionists viewed themselves as progressive Russians who would help bring about an enlightened classless society. In their desire to be fully accepted as culturally assimilated Russians, they homogenized distinctive Jewish influences into a liberal humanist agenda. While Yarros maintains that he and Spivak were religious agnostics in their youth, a common phenomenon among secular Jewish socialists, at the same time journalist Abraham Cahan recalled that Spivak clearly viewed himself as a Jew as well as a socialist, adding that "as a Jew, he had to do some thing for the Jewish future."[18] Throughout his life Spivak felt a deep sense of kinship with his fellow Jews.

Many Russian Jewish intellectuals who were transplanted to America struggled with the question of whether one could be a socialist and a Jew at the same time, as well as with broader issues regarding Jewish identity, religious observance, and connections to the larger world community,[19] but these appear to have been moot points for Spivak. In his mind they were clearly intertwined: he was a socialist *because* he was a Jew, propelled by a passionate quest for social justice and responsibility for the voiceless and underprivileged, particularly among his co-religionists—a mission that would ultimately lead to his career in medicine and tuberculosis treatment. Of course, many immigrant Jews displayed an intense commitment to progressive social and political values drawn directly or indirectly from Jewish tradition while at the same time espousing a purely secular outlook.[20] This was true of Spivak as a young man, but as the years passed his identification with the Jewish community specifically appears to have intensified, as did his connections with more traditional Jewish religious leaders and observances, even though at times he may have experienced internal conflicts.[21]

Similarly, while most Jewish intellectuals (and, not coincidentally, many of America's Jews of "German" descent) initially condescendingly viewed Yiddish, the vernacular language of the Russian Jews, as *jhargon* (an inferior dialect), Spivak the linguist—who spoke fluent Russian, Yiddish, Hebrew, German, French, and later English—positively and unambiguously viewed it as *mahma loshon* (his mother tongue). Many years later he confided to his friend Dr. Boris Bogen, "[Yiddish] is our language, the language of Jews in Diaspora. It reflects our soul and the soul of our people."[22] Of course, the Jewish legacy of multilingualism was both age-old and complex.[23] For Spivak, Yiddish helped define his identity as a Jew even as he first sought to become truly Russian and later a full American. It is telling that for the first three years of his friendship with journalist Abraham Cahan in the early 1880s, Spivak was unaware that Cahan spoke any Yiddish because of the latter's preference at the time for speaking Russian as the language of his "intellectual self."[24]

Although many Russian Jewish intellectuals, including Cahan, eventually came to appreciate Yiddish on a variety of levels, Spivak was an early unapologetic proponent. The fact that Spivak always championed Yiddish is especially noteworthy in light of the fact that the vast majority of radical Jews rejected it. As historian Ezra Mendelsohn has observed, "[M]any Russian Jewish intellectuals were, by their very nature, estranged from the Jewish masses, having abandoned both the language of the masses, Yiddish, and religious orthodoxy."[25]

Chaim Spivak's desire to be of service to humankind in general and his co-religionists in particular and his wish to prove that Jews were productive citizens sparked his membership in the famous Am Olam (Eternal People) movement, an organization of Russian Jewish emigrants who as part of the Russian "back-to-the-soil" emancipation movement hoped to found a series of Jewish farming colonies in the United States. This impetus also proved a precursor of the Kibbutz movement in Israel. According to the memoirs of Sidney Bailey, a founder of the Alliance Jewish agricultural colony located three miles from Vineland, New Jersey, Spivak had headed an Am Olam group in his hometown of Kremenschug, Russia. Thus, Spivak was one of the founding members of the short-lived but influential organization, which achieved remarkable growth in just a brief time.[26]

Am Olam was established in 1881, and a significant number of its members were Russian students like Spivak who were more interested in establishing utopian agrarian communes in America than in farming per se. About a thousand members of the Am Olam group arrived in America the following year. Chaim Spivak was among the second wave that year, part of the Kiev section led by Nicholas Aleinikoff, who later became a successful New York lawyer. Of the first five Am Olam groups of 1882, the Kremenschug, Vilna, and Odessa sections exhibited strong socialist leanings, but the Balta and Kiev groups were less doctrinaire, emphasizing instead the need to pursue lives in America based on broad principles of social justice.[27]

Strongly influenced by Russian populism and agrarian ideals and propelled by the infamous pogroms, the Am Olam groups hoped to establish a series of Jewish farm settlements in America, although a number of members had favored Ottoman Palestine over the United States, at least initially. In fact, Spivak had at first leaned toward emigration to Palestine and later recalled that he "had been occupied day and night with thundering propaganda [on behalf of Palestine]"[28] before setting off for America. One of the newspapers with which Spivak was undoubtedly familiar was the *Ha-Melitz*, edited by Alexander Zederbaum, which encouraged settlement in Palestine over America. Indeed, Spivak later became a close friend of Zederbaum's son, Dr. Adolph Zederbaum, who like Spivak ultimately chose America over Palestine and also became a physician.[29] Historian Abraham Menes has also argued that a primary aim of the Am Olam leaders was to establish a *homeland* for the Jewish people in free America and to "normalize" Jewish economic life by removing Jews from exclusive involvement in business occupations.[30]

For idealistic students, the pogroms of the early 1880s had represented not only a physical threat but a surprising rejection by the *narod*, the Russian peasant and laboring classes, whom they had supported and with whom they had hoped to usher in social change in the future. Disappointment helped fuel the mass exodus of this group of young Jews from the Russian Empire. In the words of Spivak's contemporary Abraham Cahan, "Suddenly it became clear to many young intellectual Jews that Russia was not their homeland and that a new home must be found for Jews."[31] Some, like Spivak, thought farming in the New World of America would be the answer and that an agrarian life would be the Jews' path to full social acceptance. Spivak's key role in the Jewish agricultural settlement movement in the United States will be discussed in more detail later in this chapter and in Chapter 3, but it is important to note here that his involvement in the idealistic Am Olam group was tied to his general philosophy of tearing down class barriers and improving life for the impoverished and working classes among all ethnic groups. His Am Olam connection also reflected his special affinity for Jewish agricultural undertakings and his lifelong ties to Jewish causes.

In his attraction to the ideal of Jewish farming, Spivak was a product of the ideological currents of his time. Because Russian Jews had been prevented from participating in agricultural endeavors for centuries, the Russian back-to the-land movement held special appeal for Jews. As another prominent Russian Jewish immigrant later recalled, "Farming was the ideal of intellectual Jews in those days. . . . In Jewish circles the cry then was, 'work the land.'"[32] The Russian pogroms of 1881–1882 and generally intensified discrimination against Jews graphically demonstrated that there would be little opportunity for viable Jewish life in Europe and that the Jewish intelligentsia in particular would not be able to achieve its goals of full emancipation and acceptance in Russia. Although the immediate cause of Spivak's precipitous emigration was the acute need to escape apprehension by the Russian secret police, it is likely that even without the crisis he still would have left his homeland within a short time. The Am Olam emigration to America must have appeared to Spivak and his friends to offer fresh and promising opportunities, a laboratory in which to put their ideals into practice in the benign environment of the United States. It was on his journey to America in 1882, in the Austrian town of Brody, that Spivak first met Abraham Cahan, a fellow Russian radical and later editor of the Jewish *Forward*, who became a lifelong friend.[33] When Cahan later recalled his voyage to America, he maintained that the Am Olam members he encountered on the ship "gave little thought to the doctrines of communism and socialism. They were determined only to start colonies in which life, a new kind of life for Jews, would be beautiful."[34]

Even in later years, when his reputation had grown, Spivak steadfastly refused to write his memoirs, so information on his early years comes generally from the words of friends and relatives. His close friend Isaac Rivkind, later associated with the Jewish Theological Seminary in New York City, noted that when he implored Spivak to pen his life story after he had been diagnosed with a terminal illness in 1927, Spivak again refused because he would not admit that his life had been noteworthy or extraordinary. Despite the fact that his acquaintances vehemently disagreed, Spivak told Rivkind, "I have refused Yehoash (the noted Yiddish writer and poet)

[who] was the first to ask me to write them; I have also refused Cahan (by then the famous *Forward* editor and writer)."[35]

Forced to flee Russia and despite great liberal expectations, however, like many of his cohorts Spivak was thrust into an often bewildering New World. These feelings were vividly captured by Boris Bogen, a fellow Russian immigrant and later a leading American social worker and friend of Spivak's. In his autobiography Bogen recalled, "It was terrible for me and my wife to realize that we were penniless in a strange land. I tried to find work. My halting English, my lack of experience in any trade, my bewildered look that betrayed the greenhorn, seemed to shut all doors against me. Our friends gathered about us, a generous, eager little group. But they, too, had only recently come from Moscow . . . and they were poor people—peddlers, needle workers, and 'hands' in factories and shops."[36] Similarly, Spivak's contemporary, writer Alexander Harkavy, recalled, "The plight of immigrants then was horribly bitter."[37] Part of that remarkable group of young Russian Jewish men and women who had immigrated to America in 1881 and 1882, Harkavy helped popularize Yiddish with the 1899 publication of a Yiddish-English-Hebrew dictionary, which went through many editions.

Charles Spivak did not have an easy life after his arrival. Like Bogen's friends, Spivak, too, began his American life as a factory worker in New York City, earning only six dollars a week. The theoretical discussions about "serving the people" and the exploitation of the working classes that had so preoccupied Spivak and his comrades in Russia at first became harsh realities to be confronted in America. The failure of Spivak's Am Olam commune dream and his need to resort to unaccustomed menial, back-breaking physical labor such as unloading railroad freight to earn even a meager income was an eye-opening and often bitter chapter in Spivak's life. Nearly twenty years later he recalled, "After the stormy revolutionary life in Russia and the disappointments in our ideals, we the first Russian immigrants, in our first years here in America were bereft—without a goal in life, without ideals—in a word, we felt like a teacher without pupils."[38]

Chaim Spivak experienced common immigrant feelings of loneliness, alienation, and sometimes despair upon his arrival in New York. However, like his friend Boris Bogen, with the encouragement of other Russian immigrant members of the intelligentsia and in meetings and get-togethers held in such unassuming locations as tenement rooms, cafés, and building stoops, Spivak managed to survive the adversities through his typical perseverance and eventually to acculturate and even prosper. In a 1910 article honoring writer Abraham Cahan, Spivak wrote of those early times, "I am sure that such intimate friendships rescued many from suicide."[39] Spivak had a gift for making and keeping friends, which undoubtedly helped sustain him in those difficult years. Although short of stature and somewhat stocky, Spivak was handsome; with his ready smile, thick reddish-blond hair, and a full mustache, he was a popular figure in the Russian Jewish community.

Fellow immigrants undoubtedly served as a moral support system for newer arrivals, helping them adapt through networks that helped sustain the newcomers as they made the transition from greenhorn to U.S. citizen. One of Spivak's friends who arrived in America in 1893 recalled that "[h]e [Spivak] was the first person outside of my brother, to greet me at the landing of the ship that brought me to this country."[40] The newly arrived radicals "still had at least one foot planted . . . in the rich world of Jewish social formations and group affiliations," and even if many were not religiously observant, they were still strongly influenced by "Jewish ethics, religious values, and the prophetic tradition."[41] The friendships and social gatherings also provided a forum for discussion in which the young, passionate intellectuals could argue over abstract theories and formulate new approaches, for, as Spivak later recalled, the Russian Jewish intelligentsia had brought to America "no clearly defined political, social, and economic view."[42]

Finding a job in New York City continued to be a challenge for Spivak. A popular immigrant joke that circulated among many ethnic groups at the time went something like this: I always knew the roads in America were not paved with gold, but I never imagined I would be one to pave them. Like most other Russian immigrants, Spivak spoke almost no English upon his arrival in the United States, and he possessed no practical work skills. The immigrant joke became an ironic truth for Spivak: one of his first jobs in America turned out to be that of a road paver on Broadway's Fifth Avenue. The young greenhorn also worked for a time as a typesetter for *The Jewish Messenger* in New York City and, in the late 1880s, as a farmhand and teacher at the Alliance, New Jersey, Jewish agricultural colony, supported largely by German Jewish philanthropy.[43] Spivak was not alone in his predicament, as many new immigrants endured a grinding struggle to make a living. One of his contemporaries recalled, "Not having a profession or a trade, lonely, without friends and without help, every one of us had to lead a desperate struggle for a piece of dried bread."[44]

Unable to find steady work in New York, in the fall of 1882 Spivak left to find a job in one of New England's mill towns, in a blanket factory in Winthrop, Maine. He flourished in New England, and his experiences there were chronicled in an article titled "On the Way—In an American Factory," which he published in 1884 in Russia's major radical Jewish periodical, St. Petersburg's *Voskhod* (Dawn).[45] While Spivak wrote for the publication in Russian, its audience was clearly meant to be Jewish. Because the Winthrop mill's machinery ran on waterpower, work hours were sporadic, so Charles Spivak soon moved on to another Maine factory to earn more regular wages. On the advice of a friend, he "booked a ticket to Lisbon Falls" but recalled that Winthrop "was my preparatory school for work. Before Winthrop there was only drudgery and non-contentment. There I worked peacefully and began to live."[46]

On the train to Lisbon Falls, Spivak ruminated about his former working life in New York City: "Before me passed scenes of the not-too-distant past, wandering around New York and environs. Hands were offered to anyone who was suspected of being an employer, but the soul-tearing and hope-shattering answer was 'No, Sir!'"[47] Spivak certainly did not regret leaving behind the urban congestion, filth, disease, and poor ventilation that were pervasive in New York City's immigrant tenements. Lisbon Falls in the 1880s was a typical small New England mill town and must have presented a striking contrast to the crowded streets of New York City for the young Spivak. Located near the east side of the Androscoggin River, Lisbon Falls at the time had a manufacturing population and was situated close to the Androscoggin Railroad, a branch of Maine Central. The town was rich in waterpower and was the site of the large woolen mill of the Worumbo Manufacturing Company, which had been incorporated in 1864. There was a small circulating library both in town and at the factory, surely of consequence to Spivak, an avid reader.[48] A contemporary postcard of the town pictures the Worumbo Mills in the foreground—a large brick four-story edifice, adjacent buildings, and a large smokestack dominating the edge of Lisbon Falls. Numerous small houses are visible in the background bordered by softly rolling hills, valleys, and trees. It offers a sense of what Spivak probably saw when he ventured to Lisbon Falls.

Arriving in Lisbon Falls on March 15, 1883, Spivak immediately made his way to the Worumbo Mills factory, where he was greeted by his friend sporting a bandaged hand that had been injured in a machinery accident. The old friend made light of his injury, and Spivak, with his usual wry humor, managed to turn the incident into an amusing cautionary anecdote, relating that for some time thereafter he counted his own ten fingers daily to ensure they were intact. To Spivak's surprise, he found that dozens of Russian Jewish immigrant workers, who had been sent to the site through the efforts of the Hebrew Emigrant Aid Society, were employed at the factory. Spivak was offered night work. Armed with a dinner pail with "sections like Noah's Ark for bread, butter, coffee, a glass, etc," he worked from 12:30 until 5:45 A.M., picking out burrs from wool.[49]

Unsurprisingly, night work upset Spivak's inner rhythms, and he had trouble eating and sleeping. After nearly two months of the disruptive schedule his boss took pity on the young immigrant and reassigned him to the twelve-hour day shift. During his employment at the Worumbo Manufacturing Company, Spivak encountered about sixty Jewish workers including a small number of children and women, the latter of whom received only seventy-five cents a day. He also recorded that normal wages for a male basic worker ranged from $1.12½ to $1.50 per day, low but fair.[50]

Although Spivak found the repressive and threatening atmosphere that was ever present in Russia notably absent in America, he was disturbed by the relatively low wages, sometimes dangerous work conditions, and long hours he experienced in Lisbon Falls. It also distressed him that the need for work was so desperate that no one, including himself, dared to complain openly to company officials, a surprising response considering his early radical ideology. However, he described these aspects of the work situation with his typical humor and an ironic eye, grateful for the opportunity to earn enough to sustain himself and put a little money away for the future. He was also appreciative of the easy camaraderie between the factory workers and townspeople and the integration of Jewish workers into the workforce at the American mill as well as the fact that working at the factory helped him learn to speak better English.[51] Fear and expediency may have prevented Spivak from organizing worker protests, but it is more likely that the singularities of life in America had caused him to begin to reexamine some of his vague early political ideas.

Room and board ate up much of his modest wages, and when Spivak came home at the end of the day, he often found "all the supplies, like milk, water, etc. . . . in a solid condition; frost chilled the rooms." Nevertheless, Spivak's native optimism and romantic streak inspired him to muse that if young Jewish women could be persuaded to travel to Lisbon Falls and find husbands among some of the young Jewish men in town, they "would find here healthy honest workers who are able with their callous hands to build a quiet family life, full of harmony and poetry." Spivak also looked favorably on his surroundings and found that Maine, "with its strong character, fits very well the Jewish character. This is a sober State."[52] He happily described a traditional Jewish wedding ceremony between two Jewish mill workers while he lived in the Maine town and was only saddened that the couple's parents were of necessity absent, as "[m]ay your children be raised according to Torah, the wedding canopy and good deeds is the favorite and dearest Jewish wish."[53]

Influenced by his underlying socialist ideals, Charles Spivak was proud to report that the Lisbon Falls Jewish laborers were "accepted as ready workers" and that many managed to accumulate a modest nest egg of savings and also aid relatives left behind in Europe. According to Spivak, local Jewish workers did not have an organized society during his stay, but they met often to reminisce, study English, and discuss literature; and they quickly came to the financial aid of their co-religionists when misfortune struck.[54] The young immigrant's leadership skills and magnetic personality were already evident in Lisbon Falls. A fellow immigrant later described Spivak as "the illuminating star, the heart and soul of the colony of Russian Jewish intellectual Am Olam'niks who were sent or perhaps it is better to say banished from the New York immigrant society to work in the woolen mill, far from the immigrant center in New York."[55]

In fact, his Lisbon Falls experience provided an American education of sorts for Charles Spivak, one upon which he fondly looked back. It was in the mill town that some of Spivak's new friends urged him to "talk United States!"[56] It is clear from this reference that Chaim Spivakofsky became "Charles" to his new American friends in Lisbon Falls, but he appears to have retained the surname Spivakofsky until enrolling in medical school in Philadelphia in 1887. Not only did the future physician become an eloquent speaker, but within a short time he also became an accomplished writer in the English language. Spivak's aptitude for languages certainly facilitated his rapid acquisition of English skills. Indeed, a good command of English could bring an immigrant Jew both public and political influence, a phenomenon not lost on the astute and ambitious Spivak.[57]

Not long after he left the mill town, Spivak described in glowing terms his sixteen-month stay in Lisbon Falls in a letter to the local newspaper, *The Village News*:

> It will never fade from my memory, the politeness of the kind people of your Village when conversing with me; I never perceived an offending smile on their faces while I was delivering a "speech" in the English language which was anything but English. They encouraged me by saying, "well, you talk English pretty well." Yes, Lisbon Falls was my introductory school, there I learned the language and the habits of the people of the greatest Republic on earth, every one of your citizens had a share in the good bestowed upon me. . . . In conclusion, I say in the manner of the ancient Jews of whom I am a descendant, *Shalom Aleichem*—Peace be on to you.[58]

Spivak's overt, even proud reference to his Jewish origin and affiliation is especially noteworthy. Given the fact that many Russian Jewish intellectuals studiously avoided identifying themselves as Jews whether in Russia or America,[59] it is significant that Spivak demonstrated an affirmation of his Jewish ties rather than trying to ignore or marginalize them.

Spivak's obvious admiration in the letter for the United States, "the greatest Republic on earth," is also evident and indicates that his early radical leanings were already being moderated in his adopted land. Spivak's experience in Lisbon Falls was clearly a transformative one, one of many in his event-filled life. It launched him firmly on the path to becoming an American, but one who integrated rather than discarded his immigrant background "on the way."

After leaving Maine in 1884, Spivak returned for a short time to New York City and then New Jersey, where he worked briefly as a farmhand and teacher at the Alliance agricultural colony. Fellow colonist Sidney Bailey recalled that Spivak came to Alliance as part of a larger group of "intelligentsia" in 1887 and taught adults in the colony's night school for a time.[60] Unfortunately, little detail about Spivak's stay at Alliance is known; we can only speculate that either the harsh realities of farming tarnished his agrarian idealism or that he left the colony because he felt he could be of greater benefit to humankind by entering another field. The latter notion is supported by a friend of Spivak's, who recalled that in a letter to the well-known Russian gentile utopian William Frey, a founder of the New Odessa agricultural colony, Spivak had written: "I undertook to study medicine in order to be able to serve humanity better."[61] Moreover, most Russian Jewish intellectuals only experienced short stints as workers in factories and similar laboring positions before turning to higher education, which offered them training for more prestigious professions such as law and medicine.[62]

In addition, Spivak's temperament may not have been suited to farm life, for as Joseph Brandes, who chronicled the history of the New Jersey Jewish agricultural colonies, has suggested, "[i]ronically, it was the idealistic intelligentsia who, in the long run, found the cultural paucity and drudgery of rural life the most unbearable."[63] In a letter to the Philadelphia Jewish press in 1893, Spivak, presumably drawing on his Alliance experience, acknowledged that life on a farm could indeed be dull. To prevent a mass exodus of young Jewish men from the agricultural colonies to the cities, he suggested that each settlement establish a well-stocked library, a debating society, and a lecture series to help satisfy intellectual needs.[64]

Perhaps the most important influence on Spivak's emerging philosophy and goals, as it was for many immigrant Russian Jewish intellectuals, was life in America itself. It was soon apparent to Spivak that although his first years in the United States had presented challenges, there was also unprecedented opportunity. Immigration historian Hasia Diner has maintained that the deprivation immigrants experienced in America was almost universally mild compared to that they had endured in their homelands.[65] And in regard to radical politics, as one contemporary German observer of American socialism in the early twentieth century commented, "all socialist utopias come to nothing on roast beef and apple pie."[66] Spivak's American working-class experience clearly demonstrated that despite less than optimum working conditions, being a laborer in the United States was a far cry from conditions in his Russian homeland and that the political views he had acquired in Russia were often irrelevant in his new home. In other words, the Russian model on which the Jewish radicals were raised would no longer hold.[67]

In fact, many radical Russian Jewish intellectuals were forced to remake themselves in the light of their new surroundings and circumstances.

Spivak kept in touch with a number of them his entire life and proved a loyal friend. Abe Cahan, for example, experienced a "spiritual-political" crisis in 1887, which led him to move from an ideology of anarchism to a more moderate Marxism.[68] Moreover, it was Spivak who helped guide Cahan's transformation: "A few years earlier in a letter to Dr. Chaim D. Spivak of Philadelphia, I had opened my heart and confessed my confusion."[69] Others became committed socialists and prominent leaders in the Jewish labor movement, particularly in New York City. As we shall see in Chapter 3, Spivak continued to flirt with radical political ideas for the next several years, but he was also in the process of moderating and reformulating his own ideology, and by the 1890s he had become a Social Democrat.[70] As Spivak's friend Boris Bogen put it, in America Spivak "discovered the new world. Here revolutions were not needed. Opportunities for advancement were open."[71]

These new opportunities for Spivak would germinate in Philadelphia, where he worked as a librarian and tutor to help support his medical studies. Within a short time after his arrival there, Spivak also became an acknowledged and popular leader in the city's immigrant Jewish community. In contrast to Russia, in America Spivak found a comparatively open and fluid society, where talent and ambition could project even "ordinary" men into prominence. Spivak was in Philadelphia as early as 1886. In that year he placed an advertisement in a New York Yiddish newspaper announcing that he was a "practicing teacher learned in the English, German and Hebrew languages" for hire in the City of Brotherly Love.[72] Philadelphia was only about an hour by train from the Alliance colony, and he may have commuted between the locations in the beginning. In just a few short years Spivak had crossed the divide from a young immigrant greenhorn to a Jewish American medical student, one who would someday have a profound influence on tuberculosis treatment in America and the future direction of America's Jewish community.

3

The Philadelphia Story

If the streets of New York, the textile mills in Maine, and the agricultural colonies in New Jersey provided Charles David Spivak's "elementary" education in America, the ten years he resided in Philadelphia served literally and figuratively as the time of his "higher" education—the location in which he developed his leadership skills, refined his political views, and launched his career in medicine. During Spivak's stay in Alliance, he became acquainted with the well-known New York City supporters of the East European Jewish community, Myer Isaacs and Michael Heilprin,[1] and their influence facilitated his being hired as the librarian of the Young Men's Hebrew Association (YMHA) in Philadelphia. The position with the YMHA not only helped finance Spivak's medical studies and allowed him time to study, but it also brought him to the attention of the city's more established and affluent German Jewish community. According to writer Harry Boonin, who has chronicled the history of Philadelphia's Jewish Quarter, from the first days of his arrival Spivak became a popular leader of the city's Russian Jewish colony and the most sought-after speaker among the East European immigrants.[2]

In his new home in Philadelphia's immigrant Jewish Quarter neighborhood, Spivak exhibited almost unlimited energy and excelled at what today we would call multitasking as he broadened his horizons. In 1880, before the great wave of East European immigrants arrived, there were about 15,000 Jews in Philadelphia, most from German-speaking lands. The majority of East European newcomers who swelled Jewish populations in cities around the country tended to cluster in the poorer sections of urban centers, and Philadelphia's new immigrants, including Spivak, were no exception. It was during this period in Philadelphia that Spivak first met fellow Russian immigrant Dr. Boris Bogen, later a famous social worker, who observed: "I remember that he struck me even then as an unusual character, bubbling with enthusiasm, energetic and earnest and with a lovable disposition. He was radical in his views, so were the rest, but even at that he had his own personality, his own way of thinking and doing things."[3] Still, although he was relentlessly cheerful on the outside, inwardly Spivak struggled with a number of challenges. His salary from the librarianship was meager, and he sometimes took on odd jobs such as tanning hides to make ends meet. In addition, his widowed elderly mother, who had emigrated from Russia several years after Spivak had arrived and who lived with and was supported by him at the time, suffered from severe bouts of depression and mental instability.

We are fortunate that the diary of another young Jewish physician, Dr. Michael Valentine Ball, who befriended Spivak during those early years, has recently been transcribed by Ball's grandson. It affords remarkable insight into Spivak's personality and life, including his struggles and accomplishments in Philadelphia. Ball was descended from an acculturated Jewish family of German descent, but he enjoyed his friendship with the East European–born Spivak and other members of Philadelphia's Russian Jewish colony. It appears that Ball viewed himself as a mentor of sorts to Spivak and tried to guide him toward Americanization and modification of his early radical views. Like Spivak, Ball also took a deep interest in the welfare of the poor Russian Jews in the community, especially children, offering lessons at a local Jewish "Sunday School" to "the immigrants' children in the lower end of town . . . those embryo citizens of Jewish Russian extraction."[4]

Spivak had anything but an easy life after his arrival. On May 12, 1888, Ball noted some of the more difficult aspects of Spivak's early years in Philadelphia in his diary. "In the afternoon I went to the YMHA and talked with Spivak," he wrote. "He has just placed his mother in the Insane Asylum. What a history his? How much trouble? How many things has he done to eke out a little living, and he is yet a young man, and now he fears he will go crazy too. I advised him to move from the little alley, in which he now lives, out into the bright sunshine, with friends, male and female, with whom he can talk."[5] Ball's advice proved helpful as the naturally gregarious Spivak enlarged his circle of friends.

Deborah Adel Dorfman Spivakovsky had emigrated from Russia to Philadelphia to join her only living offspring, her son "Chaimnoo" as she continued to affectionately refer to him. Ball described the circumstances that had led to the elderly Mrs. Spivakovsky's breakdown: "His mother has ever been moody, melancholy, and he has had to humour her all along. She married at 15 to one twice her age, lost 10 out of 11 children and many of her brothers and sisters, the last one but a few weeks ago, and the knowledge of whose death was kept from her until, by accident, she learned of it, which set her into a passion. She has delusions and illusions, until she became too violent to be attended at home and was taken to the Asylum."[6]

His role as the sole surviving child of a widowed, aging mother undoubtedly imposed upon Spivak a heightened sense of filial responsibility, mixed with at least some degree of guilt. While it was not unusual for Jewish immigrants to care for elderly parents, Spivak was only in his mid-twenties at the time of the incident described by Ball, and in addition to supporting and caring for Mrs. Spivakovsky he was also working his way through medical school. His experience growing up as an only child under difficult circumstances, first in Russia and later in America, may have been a key factor in his lifelong empathy for the ill and impoverished. The manner in which he reacted to the vicissitudes of life from a young age set a pattern for his life. When confronted with challenges, whether personal or professional, Spivak doggedly persevered by focusing on the tasks at hand as well as on his future goals.

Fortunately, Spivak's economic and career prospects were on the rise as he progressed in his studies, and Mrs. Spivakovsky's illness improved with treatment, which included the ministrations of a local physician named Dr. Stein. Ball noted in November 1888 that he had been introduced to

Spivak's mother at a meeting and that "[s]he is quite lucid now, though she occasionally has hysterical spells." It is interesting that the meeting was a memorial program sponsored by the "'Socialists, or Anarchists' to commemorate the deaths of the so-called Anarchists in Chicago last year."[7] While Ball seems to have attended the meeting largely out of curiosity, Spivak was there because of conviction.

Deborah Spivakovsky was well enough by 1891 to become one of the four local Jewish women who founded the Hakhnosses Orkhim Society, which established a home for wayfarers to aid the increasing number of East European Jewish immigrants arriving in the city. In 1891 the home, known as Abraham's Hotel (the biblical patriarch Abraham was known for his hospitality), was chartered, and it was supervised by Yiddish-speaking Orthodox Jewish women volunteers in the neighborhood to provide temporary shelter for newcomers on their way to a permanent location. It appears that Deborah's son, Charles Spivak, by then a full-fledged physician, treated "guests" who became ill while staying at the Lombard Street house. Spivak's mother later served as president of the Malbish Arumim (Clothe the Naked) Society, a local Jewish women's benevolent group that provided clothing to needy Jewish children in the neighborhood.[8]

Michael Ball's diary also provides valuable glimpses into Spivak's evolving political views as well as his years as both a medical student and later a physician. Spivak's YMHA job provided the opportunity to debate political and social issues with fellow immigrants and other medical students. Ball's first diary reference to Spivak occurred on September 24, 1887, when he noted, "I went to the YMHA and read *The Exponent* and then talked to the librarian, Mr. Spivakofsky, who is now studying medicine."[9] On November 13 that same year he wrote, "I had a very interesting talk with Spivakofsky on 'Free Speech,' etc."[10] A year later Ball attended another lecture and ran into "a young lady friend of Spivak, whom I accompanied to the library, where he was waiting for her. She is an enthusiastic Anarchist, but I think I raised some doubts in her mind."[11] It is possible that the lady in question was Jennie Charsky, a Russian Jewish immigrant who was known for her early radical views and whom Spivak married in 1893. Spivak and Ball continued their political discussions as time went on, and one evening, when Ball's regular obstetrics lecture class was cancelled, he "went to the YMHA and talked until 11:30 with Spivak on Labor, Land, and Capital questions."[12]

In the fall of 1887, Spivak began a three-year course of medical studies at Philadelphia's Jefferson Medical College, founded in 1824. Spivak had come in contact with such Jewish notables as the famous German-born Jewish jurist Mayer Sulzberger, Dr. Solomon Solis-Cohen, and Dr. Sabato Morais through the Alliance colony; and these men or others like them in Philadelphia may have contributed moral and financial support toward his studies. Solis-Cohen was a prominent local Philadelphia Jewish doctor who had graduated from Jefferson Medical College in 1883. The Sephardic Reverend Dr. Sabato Morais was the well-known leader of Philadelphia's traditional synagogue, the Spanish Portuguese Mikveh Israel, the oldest and most prestigious congregation in Philadelphia. Spivak's capabilities and personality no doubt impressed members of the established Jewish community, and his friend Victor Yarros noted that Spivak had entered Jefferson Medical College "with the aid and support of some friends."[13] Perhaps the rapidly Americanizing Spivak served as a Russian Jewish success story to be held up as an example for newer immigrants. In any case, Spivak's essays and letters were frequently printed in Philadelphia's *Jewish Exponent*, a newspaper founded by members of the city's Jewish elite to help, in part, Americanize the Russian immigrants.[14]

Ball was a class ahead of Spivak, and his diary gives us a good idea of the curriculum at Jefferson Medical School, which included lectures in such subjects as obstetrics, gastroenterology, and "neuralgia," as well as experience in surgical clinics and a regular chemical laboratory class. At the close of the Civil War, medical education in America was generally informal and courses superficial. As the decades passed, in response to public pressure and the medical profession itself, course work became more comprehensive and scientific, and many schools incorporated medical research and clinical experience into the study program.[15] Most medical schools at the turn of the twentieth century still had less exacting standards than we would expect today, but Jefferson Medical College was considered one of the better institutions. Indeed, in a famous and highly critical report on the state of medical education in the United States and Canada published by the educator Dr. Abraham Flexner of New York in 1910, Jefferson was lauded as one of three institutions that had established its own excellent teaching hospital for senior medical students. The famous "Flexner Report," as it was termed, helped spark a revolution in medical education in the United States by 1920.[16]

At Jefferson Medical College, Spivak and Ball were exposed to a variety of subjects taught by a number of qualified local physicians including Dr. Solis-Cohen, who was the clinical lecturer on medicine while Spivak was a student, and both received hands-on training in local clinics and hospitals. The friendship between Spivak and Ball was fostered by their shared interest in medicine, the Jewish immigrant community, and politics. In 1889 Ball traveled to Germany, considered the most advanced country in the world in the area of medicine at the time and where he had a number of relatives, to pursue graduate studies in medicine. Studying in Germany was a common practice among young German Jewish doctors during the era. In Germany, Michael Ball worked under the eminent bacteriologist Robert Koch, whose discovery of the tubercle bacillus in 1882 revolutionized the understanding of the dread disease, formerly considered hereditary for the most part. Although both Ball and Spivak had very full schedules, they continued to keep in touch while Ball was in Europe through correspondence that still included discussions of political philosophy: "I received a letter from Spivak, who is busy with his [medical] studies . . . he must leave off his Socialistic-Anarchistic ideas to which he still clings. The world is not yet ripe for them. And to force them upon the populace would be contrary to the principles of the Socialists who do not want to be forced themselves."[17]

Despite his very busy days and evenings, throughout his stay in Philadelphia Spivak also took a central role in the Russian Jewish community. Soon after his arrival, Spivak was asked to give a lecture for the leading Russian immigrant group, the Russian Jewish Hebrew Literature Society, for he was equally at home in Hebrew, Yiddish, and the Russian language. His gift for humor and his speaking abilities so impressed reporters from the local newspaper, *The Jewish Exponent*, that he was invited to contribute articles to the periodical. Spivak remained a frequent writer for the publication for many years.[18] In March 1888 Ball had attended a meeting of the Russian Jewish Tourgeniff Literary Club, where he listened to a lecture in English on Benjamin Franklin given by a local Jewish attorney. Following the lecture, "Spivakofsky, who is one of the leaders of this club, gave, in Russian, an extract from [journalist] Kenneth's article in *The Century* on 'Russian Prisons.'"[19] Spivak was also the primary founder of the Russian American Organization (RAO). In 1889 he invited his old Am Olam friend, Nicholas Aleinikoff, to give a public lecture to the group. Aleinikoff, by then a prominent figure in New York's East European Jewish community, spoke on "The Socialist Position of the Russians and Its Impact on America,"[20] an appropriate topic given Spivak's close ties to socialism and the Russian Jewish community.

While employed as the YMHA librarian and as a medical student, Spivak also found the time to teach Hebrew for the Hebrew Education Society along with his newfound good friend Reverend Sabato Morais. Morais, minister-*chazan* (cantor) at the Orthodox Mikveh Israel congregation, was Spivak's senior by nearly forty years. Although committed to traditional Judaism, Morais was a force for Americanization in the lives of the new immigrants, including Spivak. In a speech before his own congregants, Morais once maintained that "[w]ith the spangled banner of liberty in on one hand, and the law of Horeb[21] in the other, we will continue faithful citizens of this glorious republic."[22]

Despite his radical leanings, Spivak retained friendships with Orthodox and traditional rabbis, a pattern later evidenced in Denver. These relationships may have helped him reconcile tensions among religion, politics, and science that surfaced at intervals in his life such as his support of autopsy, which was in most cases in opposition to traditional Jewish law. Spivak and Morais sometimes traveled to New Jersey agricultural colonies to offer encouragement to the farmers. At one such meeting at the Carmel Colony, Morais spoke, and Spivak elucidated and translated Morais's remarks for the largely Yiddish- and Russian-speaking audience.[23]

Perhaps in response to Ball's advice to spend more time among friends, Spivak also took part in local Philadelphia amateur theater through the Russian dramatic circle. As an added bonus, he probably honed his speaking abilities through acting. In October 1888 the twenty-seven-year-old Spivak played the male lead in Gogol's *The Marriage* opposite the seventeen-year-old leading lady Jennie Charsky, who became Spivak's wife five years later. *The Jewish Exponent* reviewed the play, which was performed in "faultless and genuine Russian"; while Spivak was judged adequate for the role, Jennie was lauded as highly effective and "vivacious."[24]

Once again, Ball's diary provides an insider's view of key events in Spivak's life. Ball recorded one of the performances of the play in his diary. In November 1888 Ball noted that he and a friend attended a performance of a Russian play in which Spivak took part, "his first appearance on the stage. . . . After the play, we made our way to the stage, and behind the scenes, congratulated Spivak and heard of its success. It is the first Russian play, played by Russians and in Russian, a language few perfectly understand, much less speak, in this city." Always the moralist, Ball revealed his somewhat condescending outlook toward the Yiddish-speaking East European Jews when he continued: "I intend to witness soon some of the jargon, or 'Yiddish' plays that are enacted here quite often and that are, no doubt, funny. I think that a great deal can be done with the drama among our co-religionists, spreading moral truths, giving them a place for innocent enjoyment and social meet."[25] Charles Spivak remained active in the Russian Dramatic Club until he and Jennie left for Denver in 1896, the year the group disbanded.[26]

The former Chaim Dovid Spivakovsky, who had shortened and Americanized his name to Charles David Spivak, graduated with honors from Jefferson Medical College in 1890. The final step involved the testimony of Dr. Lewis W. Steinbach of Philadelphia, who certified on February 21, 1890, that "Mr. Chas. D. Spivak is 28 years of age, of good moral character, and by April 1890, will have read the various branches of Medicine at least three years." At the bottom of the certificate Spivak signed his name as Charles D. Spivak in his distinctive handwriting, attesting that "[t]he undersigned hereby makes application for examination for the degree of M.D., having complied with all the requirements."[27] Steinbach, who was a decade older than Spivak, was also part of the circle of Jewish doctors in Philadelphia. He, too, was a graduate of Jefferson Medical College and in 1894 served as a professor of clinical and operative surgery at the Philadelphia Polyclinic. Steinbach probably met Spivak at the YMHA, in which both were active.[28]

Shortly after returning from his year of study in Germany, on April 2, 1890, Dr. Michael Ball attended the graduation ceremonies of the newly minted Dr. Spivak and their mutual friend, German-born Dr. Ludwig Loeb. In describing the event, Ball related, "quietly stirring myself and ordering two bouquets for Spivak and Loeb, I entered the Academy of Music and seated myself on the stage, meeting many of the graduates and classmates of last year."[29] Charles David Spivak was now officially a qualified physician, and his diploma would serve as a passport into mainstream American life.

Just two days later, Dr. Ball joined Spivak and his mother for the Passover Seder. Ball's description of the evening gives a vivid firsthand account of the obstacles the young physician had encountered and what challenges still lay ahead. Ball recounted that "Spivak called in the morning and invited me up to his house for the Passover meal. . . . I dressed for the evening and took a car for Spivak's. They were waiting for me. Spivak, his mother, a friend of his, with his wife, his aunt and several of her children, and one or two others were there. His mother was looking very well, and was very glad to see me. She had undergone the whole strain that Spivak had in his examination, and, as her son says, was entitled to a diploma as much as he was." Spivak, an early agnostic, "led the service and sang the songs very well. It was a double rejoicing for him and his mother, for now he had virtually crossed the Red Sea, but of student life and its slavery, and he was a free man, free to make his living now with a handiwork that he could make it with but he is yet to go through the wilderness of that time that hangs on a young practitioner's hands and wait patiently before he can say he is self supporting."[30]

The passage also reveals the concern for others that seems to have formed the core of Charles Spivak's personality. Ball continued, "He [Spivak] has had a tough time of it. This winter, his aunt and four little children, her mother, and a young man came to him with about 2 Rubles in their pockets, and, out of his barely-sufficient-to-live means, he had to keep them the whole winter. Now the woman, a comely and strong woman, is making $7 a week by serving, but oh, how she must work to do it."[31]

Spivak's sensitivity is also revealed in an amusing story about the relationship between Spivak and his mother, Deborah, retold by Max Shulman—later president of the Zionist organization of Chicago, with whom Spivak shared a lifelong commitment to Zionism. According to Shulman the incident was related to him by a Dr. J. Gartenstein, an "eye-witness to the scene," which occurred about 1895. Shulman recounted:

> After several years of hard struggle, Spivak was graduated at the Jefferson College and became active in Jewish life as a leader and teacher. At one meeting where he was announced to lecture, his old mother, dressed in an old fashioned shawl, wearing a "*Sheitel*" [traditional Jewish wig] came to the meeting but would not be admitted. After making a disturbance, she finally gained admittance, rushed up to the platform where her son was lecturing and exclaimed, "Chaim, they would not admit your mother—leave the hall immediately." Chaim stopped his lecture, walked over to his mother, embraced her

> affectionately, kissed her tenderly and escorted her to the platform, seated her calmly and then continued with his lecture.[32]

In May 1890 Dr. Ball, who appears to have been working in a local clinic or hospital, was able to report, "I received a letter from Dr. Spivak. He has an office now and has made $5 in 23 days, but that is good."[33] Spivak opened his first medical practice in a historic house at 338 Spruce Street in Philadelphia's Jewish Quarter. It was one of many attached narrow, red brick townhouses on the street without a front yard, which merely featured several steps at the front door that led directly to the sidewalk. Characteristically, Spivak also spent much of his time offering his services to poor immigrant Jews with Dr. Ludwig Loeb, with whom he opened a dispensary called the Maimonides Clinic in June 1891 on Philadelphia's Lombard Street. The undertaking was apparently initiated at the suggestion of their mutual friend Michael Ball, who noted in his diary in early July, "Loeb and Spivak have arranged it so that a dispensary will be opened down in the lower end of town under the auspices of the Jewish Community. It was my idea. I gave it to Loeb and he worked it out."[34]

Medical dispensaries were common in many cities around the country in the late nineteenth and early twentieth centuries and helped provide medical treatment to the urban poor, often immigrants, who otherwise would have been unable to afford the services of physicians or the cost of medications. As medical historian Charles Rosenberg has observed, the dispensary reflected "an important aspect of [both] medicine and philanthropy in the 19th-century city,"[35] and these two central features of Spivak's life found expression in his personal involvement in such an undertaking. The two young immigrant doctors—Spivak and Loeb—provided medical care, surgical treatment, and home visits, when necessary, to about fifty poor Jewish patients each week. In addition, patients could purchase drugs at the dispensary for only twenty cents per prescription. In 1893 the clinic relocated to Spruce Street, the street that served as the location for Spivak's first and second medical offices and homes.[36] Spivak's second home and office was a smaller townhouse but more centrally located, perhaps reflecting the fact that the thirty-two-year-old doctor was developing a fine reputation that resulted in a growing practice. However, money was never plentiful for Spivak, as throughout his life he generally treated impoverished patients.

A colleague of Spivak's recalled that "as a practitioner, first in Philadelphia, and later in Denver, he [Spivak] was a busy and painstaking gastroenterologist. His reputation, coupled with his good nature, won and kept for him many patients. . . . In spite of his busy practice, Dr. Spivak, from the very outset, found time to do investigative [research] work."[37] Although only in his early thirties, in 1893 he was appointed chief of the clinic for gastrointestinal disease, his specialty, at the Philadelphia Polyclinic. His first technical medical writings appeared in New York and local medical journals as early as 1895 when he still resided in Philadelphia, but his first article in the prestigious *Journal of the American Medical Association* (JAMA), titled "Rest—A Neglected Factor in the Treatment of Gastro-Intestinal Disorder," was not published until July 1898, two years after he had moved to the Queen City of Denver.[38] However, Spivak likely formulated his ideas for the essay while still in Philadelphia. Reading his medical articles today, it is clear that. Spivak's felicitous writing style extended to his medical papers.

His graduation from medical school and growing prominence in the Philadelphia medical and general communities apparently did not deter Spivak from Jewish community work. His interest in Jewish farming continued, and he became a frequent contributor to a variety of Jewish periodicals. In August 1890 he was chosen president pro tem of the Jewish Alliance of America. Coverage of a mass meeting for the new organization appeared in *The Philadelphia Inquirer* on August 11, 1890. The newspaper reported that delegates from local Jewish organizations had met to discuss assistance for Russian Jews being driven out of Russia by the czar's new edicts and that the object of the Jewish Alliance was to promote "the welfare of Russian Jews."[39] The organization's initial founding meeting was actually held at Dr. Spivak's first medical office at 338 Spruce Street. A letter preserved from Spivak to Morais, dated August 14, 1890, mentioned that early meeting at Spivak's house and invited Morais to join him for a follow-up meeting where "a plan of organization will be laid before the meeting." Spivak ended the letter by saying, "We hope you will grace us with your presence."[40]

The Jewish Alliance had been founded as a national organization by the young doctor and another Russian-born Jewish immigrant, attorney Bernard Harris, to assist Jewish immigrants once they arrived in the United States.[41] Spivak viewed the challenge of dealing with the tide of Jewish immigration as an opportunity to bring all Jews in America together to support the newcomers. At the time, Spivak observed, "The American, the German, the Hungarian, the Portuguese and Russian Hebrews have come together for the first time; they have found the platform which unites them all."[42]

Spivak and Harris shared a common background as East European immigrants who had begun to enter the American mainstream through their chosen professional fields. Despite their evolving acculturation and Americanization, both young men (they were just a year apart in age, Harris having been born in Vilna in 1862) had a passionate commitment to their fellow immigrants, both were contributing journalists, and both had developed ties to the city's German Jewish leaders such as Mayer Sulzberger, one of America's leading Jewish attorneys and judges.

In an article written for *The Jewish Exponent*, Spivak outlined the purpose and justification for the organization and maintained, "There has never been a society in the United States organized for the purpose of [Jewish] colonization. The Jewish Alliance of America is such a one."[43] He observed that East European immigration to the United States showed no signs of abating, as Russian persecution of Jews remained ongoing, and predicted that the continued swelling of the Jewish immigrant population in large urban cities of the East would exacerbate nativism and anti-Semitism. "The cry 'America for Americans' is the danger signal," he warned.[44] While he did not propose turning all immigrants into farmers, Spivak clearly saw a partial solution to some of the immigrants' problems through agriculture: "What we mean by our plan of colonization is to get as many away from the large cities as can be encompassed by our means. The settling of ten families upon ten farms in one year means ten families away from the gutters, from the basket and from the sewing machine."[45]

In an attempt to address the critics of Jewish colonization, Spivak utilized the arguments of the American Jewish elite. In 1890 agrarian idealism was still very much a part of American thought, despite the fact that in reality the United States, including the West, had become increasingly urbanized and industrialized.[46] Farming was not only seen as a noble ideal, but for men like Morais, Solis-Cohen, and Sulzberger it seemed a positive solution for removing Jews from overcrowded urban ghettos and at the same time diffusing anti-Semitism. As Joseph Brandes has observed, support for the Jews as an agricultural people became very popular among leaders of the era's American Jewish establishment.[47] Not long after Spivak's article appeared in *The Jewish Exponent*, the even better-known *American Israelite* (Cincinnati), edited by Isaac Mayer Wise, reported that Dr. Solis-Cohen had also maintained that "[o]ne of the principal objects of the [Jewish] Alliance was to make farmers of the Jews, who crowded the cities."[48]

If Spivak was influenced by Russian populism and its idealized view of the serfs as the most productive members of Russian society, he was attracted as well by the American agrarian myth. In August 1887, while a medical student, he had visited the Jewish agricultural colony at Vineland, New Jersey, and happily reported that "despised and persecuted even now in almost every country of the Old World, these [Jewish] descendants are now free men, equal citizens and honest tillers of the soil."[49] It has been demonstrated that a number of Russian Jewish intellectuals retreated to pastoral themes in reaction to urbanization.[50] The concept of the individual farmer as the moral, independent base upon which America would stand, however, was an old one and had been espoused by Thomas Jefferson and Benjamin Franklin in the early days of the Republic.[51]

When Spivak called for the Jews "to take up the plow and hoe, the trade of [their] forefathers," and maintained along with Prince Kropotkin, a Russian anarchist theorist and writer, that "despite industrialization, agriculture should still be considered a stronghold of the Malthusian theory,"[52] Spivak—at least in his rhetoric—drew upon the Russian and American strains that influenced his thinking. Kropotkin believed that placed in a "natural state," without the interference of government, people would work cooperatively, and thus his theories could be used to support the communal agrarian colonies that so appealed to Spivak.

In their view of Jewish colonization—particularly in the western states—as at least a partial solution to the problem of the staggering influx of Jewish immigration,[53] Spivak and his supporters were once again unwittingly echoing the prescient sentiments of an early American spokesperson for the agrarian ideal. In the early 1780s Hector St. John Crevecoeur, an intellectual gentleman farmer, had declared that the West would become an "asylum of freedom . . . the refuge of distressed Europeans."[54] Crevecoeur was not, of course, referring to Russian Jews, but the concept of the farmer as a free, independent, and valuable individual was easily adapted by Jewish proponents of agricultural settlement. Although they lived a century apart, both Spivak and Crevecoeur viewed the American West as the "last frontier," where an abundance of land could support numerous immigrants. Spivak was certainly reflecting the idea, popular at the time in many radical Jewish circles, that physical labor and agrarianism were more noble than engaging in commerce.

Spivak never ascribed the failure of so many Jewish colonies either to the farmers themselves or to farming as an occupation but rather to the fact that the colonies had received inadequate financial backing from the Jewish establishment to buy proper tools, machinery, and other necessary items.[55] He wrote of the western colonies, for example, that "[t]hey were not conducted on business principles, the money came always too late."[56] It is ironic that Spivak, who generally idealized farming in his writings, recognized the need for mechanization, business skills, and adequate capital as a prerequisite to successful farming. It demonstrates perhaps, as did his later work with the JCRS, that Spivak was at once an idealist and a pragmatist.

Sometime between the fall of 1890 and the beginning of 1891, the emphasis of the Jewish Alliance of America shifted from Jewish colonization to the unification of the established German Jewish community and Russian Jews already in America as a means of assisting the new tides of East European immigrants. To this end, a national convention was held in Philadelphia on February 15, 1891, at the YMHA, with hundreds of delegates attending from all over the United States.[57] Delegates discussed such issues as providing aid to the immigrants, how best to educate them as to their duties as American citizens, and how to help them become self-supporting. Once again, emphasis was placed on settling the new immigrants in areas of the West, away from crowded urban ghettos. At this convention Spivak delivered the major address and was elected a vice president of the national organization. Simon Muhr, a German Jewish philanthropist from Philadelphia, was elected president.[58]

Like many acculturating immigrants, Charles Spivak continued to struggle to balance his American, Russian, and Jewish sensibilities. Surely it was not mere coincidence that the stage for the convention sported numerous American flags as well as posters in Hebrew with appropriate slogans and biblical quotes,[59] probably Spivak's handiwork. A year later the group combined with other Jewish organizations to form the American Committee for Ameliorating the Condition of the Russian Refugees. Both groups disappeared into oblivion within a short time as responsibility for the immigrants was taken over primarily by the Baron de Hirsch Fund.[60]

In the fall of 1891 Spivak left for postgraduate work in Europe. He stopped briefly in Paris and then went on to Germany, where he attended the University of Berlin to enhance his medical knowledge—not a common practice among East European immigrant physicians. Given Spivak's modest financial situation, it is possible that his studies in Europe were financed by an affluent Jewish sponsor in Philadelphia. The Philadelphia *Public Ledger* noted his departure: "Dr. Charles D. Spivak, who is well known as a Vice President of the Jewish Alliance of America, sailed for Europe last week. He expects to remain there several months, devoting his time to studying new developments in medicine."[61] By late May or early June 1892 Spivak was back in Philadelphia because he is recorded as having delivered a baby there in June.[62]

As Charles Spivak became established as a prominent doctor and community leader, his political ideas evolved into a moderate socialism that was more congruent with his new American circumstances. The radical politics of his youth were undergoing refinement and modification. In his memoirs, Russian radical Leon Kobrin recalled being treated by Spivak in the early 1890s for an injury he had sustained while working in a local sweatshop, a graphic reminder of the frequent perils of industrialization for common laborers. Spivak treated Kobrin's hand and also gave him a strong dose of advice about radical politics, advising him that anarchism was impractical and too focused on a nebulous future and suggesting that Kobrin should reconsider his views. "In the meantime," Spivak counseled in Russian, "we should ask the Social Democrats to help us improve conditions of life for mankind that lives in today's society. . . . [Y]es, dear young man, what's worse is not better, as your anarchists babble, but what's better is better. Familiarize yourself with the literature of the Social Democrats."[63]

The three young Jewish doctors—Spivak, Loeb, and Ball—remained friends, and in August 1892 Ball reported that "[w]e have formed a society to study Philosophy. Spivak, Miss Jennie Charsky (Spivak's intended), Dr. Loeb, myself, and one or two others."[64] While Michael Ball had criticized Spivak's early radical politics, the friends shared an idealistic commitment to social justice for humankind as well as a passion for intellectual discourse. Ironically, Ball, himself committed to various social causes, described Spivak in his diary as "idealistic" but also as "[w]ise in language, literature, political economy, etc."[65] He was somewhat conflicted and skeptical about an idea Spivak had shared with him for a new project: "Spivak has a scheme in view. He is full of schemes, but he never carries them out. He envisions a lecture course with stereopticon views, for the poor people free of charge, on travel, literature, art, etc., he and I and others to start. I am in with the movement heart and soul and hope we can accomplish it."[66]

Whether the lecture series came to fruition is unknown, but by the next year Spivak and Jennie Charsky, whom he had known at least since she was a teenager, were married. Like her new husband, Jennie Charsky was an East European Jewish immigrant. She was born on September 24, 1871, in Poltava, Russia, the daughter of Saul and Chaya Shamus Charsky, who passed away when her children were still young. Jennie arrived in America as a teenager, followed by her two younger sisters, to join their father, a member of the Rosenheyn Jewish agricultural colony in New Jersey near Alliance.[67] We do know that Jennie was well-known to Spivak by 1888 when the seventeen-year-old (ten years younger than Spivak) acted opposite him in the previously noted Russian plays. Jennie was animated, mercurial, intellectually gifted, and determined or stubborn, depending on who was describing her. She was also highly unconventional in her politics and lifestyle as a young woman in her late teens and early twenties. Contemporary pictures reveal an attractive young woman of short stature, a slim figure, and with a cropped, boyish haircut. Spivak was highly attracted to the intense, energetic young woman, with whom he shared interests in politics, philosophy, literature, theater, and Jewish agricultural endeavors. Jennie was also a budding writer who later authored many newspaper and magazine articles, a play, and a volume of poems.

Something of an intellectual bluestocking, Jennie pursued her higher education at a variety of universities. First, she studied at West Chester Normal School, a teacher's training institute near Philadelphia, beginning classes there in September 1889. It is probable that Spivak either helped finance her education himself, a course Ball alluded to in his diary, or that Charles helped Jennie make connections with members of Philadelphia's elite like Mayer Sulzberger, who could be persuaded to aid a promising East European immigrant. A letter from Spivak to Sabato Morais in December 1890 sheds light on the subject. In the letter Spivak asks Morais to provide a recommendation to the Normal School on behalf of a young Russian Jewish woman who "desires to follow in the path of Miss Charsky." He explains that Jennie Charsky had come to an agreement with the school's superintendent that allowed her to repay her tuition fees after she graduated and began teaching.[68] Normal schools were generally two-year institutions that concentrated on instruction in education, teaching techniques, and classroom management; and many potential teachers honed their professional skills in model or "practice" schools associated with those institutions. Although limited in scope, the normal schools, which welcomed the attendance of intelligent women who had completed a high school course, provided higher education for women in an era during which university opportunities for women were still limited and created "an environment where women could blossom."[69]

Probably influenced by Spivak, in 1891 Jennie left the normal school to enroll as a biology major at the University of Pennsylvania, but she found that she was not welcomed by the male students. The following year she took another daring step, enrolling as a law student at Cornell University in Ithaca, New York, but she left after one semester to marry Charles Spivak. At Cornell Jennie, who used her formal name Evgenya Lazarevna Charsky, successfully completed classes in contracts and torts, among several other subjects.[70]

Ball was well acquainted with "Miss Charsky," whom he had encountered many times during his friendship with Charles Spivak. Jennie apparently clung to her radical views longer and more strongly than her fiancé had. Ball did not seem much taken with Jennie at first and observed in his diary: "Spivak is very fond of Miss Charwoskey [Charsky], loves her dearly."[71] Spivak and Jennie Charsky, whose Jewish name was Gittel, were married at B'nai Jacob synagogue on March 27, 1893, by the Russian-born Rabbi Chaim Shraga Brodsky, with whom Spivak shared a commitment to Jewish values, Zionism, and moderate socialist views. B'nai Jacob was located only a block from Spivak's home, so he likely attended services there, at least on occasion. Ball attended the wedding ceremony and wrote:

> The bride is embarrassed. Spivak is glad. Of all the wedding ceremonies [I have attended] this was the most curious. It was like Catherine and Petruchio in a sense, for I think Miss Charwoskey did not want to undergo the ceremony in the least. The friends, many of them radical in their views, laughed and giggled . . . while the Rabbi . . . quickly

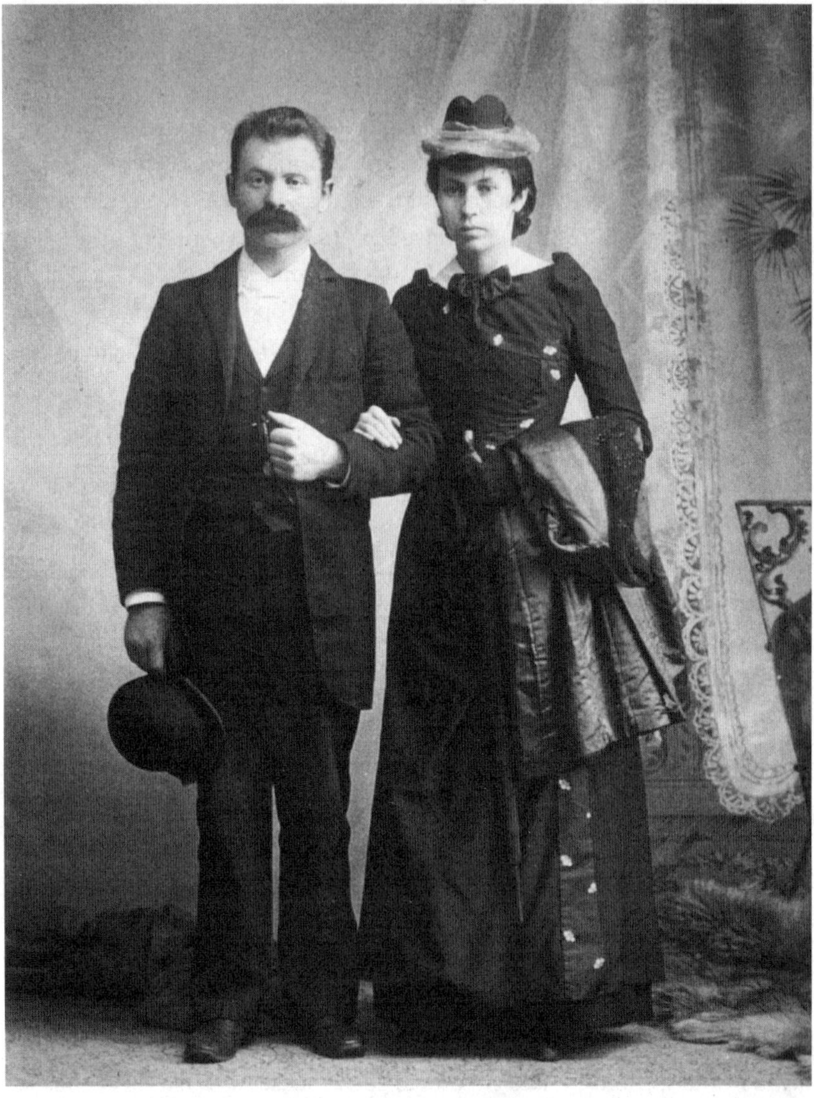

Studio portrait of Dr. Charles David Spivak with his fiancée, Jennie, Philadelphia, September 1892. The picture was taken the day before Jennie left to attend college at Cornell University. Courtesy, Charlesa Wolfe Feinstein.

mumbled out the religious and legal formula. . . . The ring was put on. A general kissing of the Bride and Groom followed, and they were legally man and wife, what they had been by mutual consent before. I

> was glad of this legal formula, for I feared that she would leave Spivak, wrecking his life and her own. She is a willful girl, full of radical ideas without a firm basis. Marriage and religion are all mockery in her eyes, and yet, she is only 22 or 23 years old. Spivak has indulged her as a spoilt child, educated her in every whim. She has studied law a short while, then a short term at the University, etc. Now, he at least, will have rest. What their life will be, I do not know. He needs a woman that he will have to direct.[72]

Ball, still a bachelor, does not appear to have been completely accurate in his assessment of the marriage because subject to the test of time, Jennie and Charles seem in many ways to have been well-suited soul mates. Certainly, Spivak remained devoted to Jennie, or "Gittele," as he affectionately called her, throughout his life and was ahead of his time in his efforts to support his wife's educational and creative aspirations. Spivak seems to have treated women as equals and had a female physician working alongside him in the dispensary. A photograph taken of Spivak and Jennie in 1892 bears an inscription on the back in Spivak's handwriting that reads: "Taken on Monday, Sept. 26, 1892, the day of the departure of the lady of my heart for the Cornell University." As an indication of his devotion, the word "my" is underscored four times. Jennie and Charles appear in the photograph standing with arms linked, and Jennie's Russian name, Luba, is penned in under her picture.

However, Ball presciently seems to have realized early on that Jennie's volatile personality might continue to be a challenge to Spivak in the future. It is possible that the highly individualistic Jennie sometimes chafed at playing Pygmalion to Spivak's Galatea. Several letters addressed to Dr. Spivak in the early 1920s indicate that when Jennie was in her late forties, she experienced a period of mental instability that required her to be hospitalized. Spivak stood by her at that time, as he had earlier with his mother under similar circumstances, until the crisis passed.[73] It is clear that with the advent of her marriage in 1893 and motherhood as time went on, as was the case with her husband, Charles, Jennie moderated her more radical political views as she matured and became even more active in the Jewish and general communities.

Before her marriage, Jennie had taught English to Jewish newcomers in Philadelphia and had founded a group called the Daughters of Israel, which worked to assist poor Russian immigrants.[74] The newlywed Mrs.

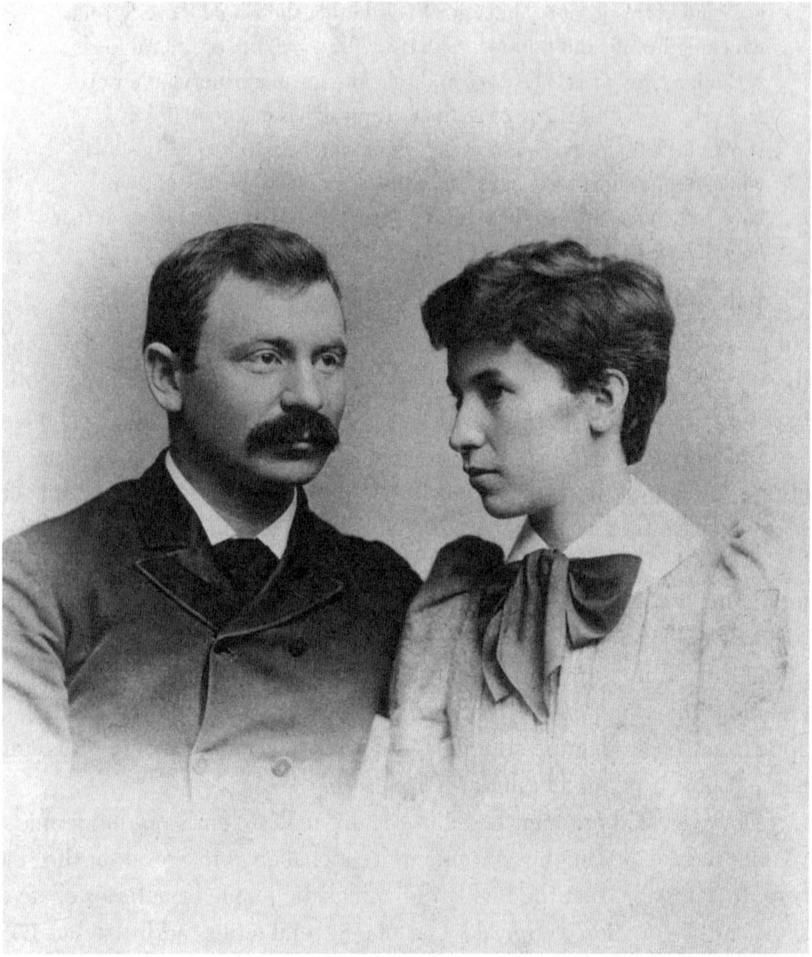

Portrait of Dr. Charles David and Jennie Charsky Spivak, 1893. Courtesy, Charlesa Wolfe Feinstein.

Spivak continued her interest in the newcomers. Ball, who became active in settlement work with immigrants and minority groups, noted that "with others, we have started a girls' club, mostly Russian girls of 16 and over. It is quite prosperous. Mrs. Spivak was made President. I visit them once a week. They have reading and singing classes, and a great deal is expected of this club."[75] In August 1893 Ball ran into Jennie at the Alliance Jewish agricultural colony, in which both took an interest.[76]

Barely nine months after their marriage, Jennie and Charles became the parents of their first child, a son named David. Once again their good friend Dr. Michael Ball was present at the family celebration, serving as the "Koom" (godfather) at the *bris milah*, the Jewish circumcision ceremony. Ball recorded at length the details of the happy event and celebratory meal, which sent the household into a great uproar:

> Spivak is a father and I presided at the circumcision of the child. The house was in a flurry. Mrs. Spivak was excited and nervous, and Spivak himself was all upset, hardly knowing what to do or say. Mrs. Spivak, Sr., is so happy, that she could do nothing but talk. Two physicians, friends of mine, were present. The grandmother, who was my partner, takes the child on a cushion, brings it to the operating room, the parlor, and hands it to me. I take it and give it to the Rabbi, who pronounces a Hebrew prayer. Then, setting himself on the table, he takes the child in his lap. The physician now makes the circumcision, one cut and it is over. The father looks on, faint[s] almost, to see his first child, his own, bleed.[77]

Ball continued to describe the hectic scene at the celebration:

> The Rabbi says another prayer, the child is given to me, and I return it to the grandmother . . . who takes it back to the anxious mother, who now fondles her darling with caresses and tears. Congratulations are now handed around. The father is still in a stupor. . . . Dinner is served, but the old grandmother is excited and the Rabbi is hungry and the hired girl is missing and one delay after another until the herring comes. The Rabbi says the prayer over the twisted bread. After the herring comes the soup, but a spoon is missing here, a fork there, and this one is not served, and that one is forgotten. The soup over, amidst the chatter of the grandmother and a discourse between the philosopher and the Rabbi on circumcision, the meat comes in, with pickles and dessert. The father has a case to attend to and off he rushes.[78]

Spivak proved to be a doting father to David and two more children born to the Spivaks: Deena, who arrived on February 21, 1895, in Philadelphia, and the baby of the family, Ruth, born in Denver in 1902. Propelled in part by their growing family, the Spivaks moved to a townhouse at 529 Pine Street in May 1895, which also served as Spivak's last office in Philadelphia. It was a large home, and the Spivaks took in several

Russian-born immigrant friends as boarders—probably to supplement the family's income, as Dr. Spivak often struggled to make a living in the early years.[79]

As Ball's description of the circumcision ceremony demonstrates, Charles and Jennie Spivak—the early radical revolutionaries and religious skeptics—welcomed their new son into the world with a traditional *bris*, the same ways Jewish males had been ushered into the Jewish people since the biblical recording of the ritual beginning with the biblical patriarch Abraham. No more mention of the Spivaks appears in Ball's diary until February 25, 1896, when he observed, "Spivak has had to go to Colorado with his wife. At first he thought of turning his work to me, but on more consideration, thought not. I have opened up a small office downtown as an experiment."[80] Just a few weeks later, however, the circumstances had changed:

> What is one man's poison is another's food. Spivak found that his wife was ailing, so he decided to go to Colorado and asked me to take his work. He makes about $200 a month, but [it] is awfully hard work and all sorts. I will have to take his home. I tried to persuade him not to go, to let his wife go, but he decided otherwise. And so it is arranged for this month sometime. I have given up all ideas of succeeding where I am, although I had made a few cents, but just enough to pay for my wash.[81]

Charles Spivak's departure from Philadelphia left a great void in the city, both because of his growing reputation as a fine medical clinician, researcher, and sensitive physician and also because of the key role he had played in the Jewish community. Ball mentions, "My taking Spivak's place necessitated my joining lodges, etc., which I have already done, B'nai B'rith, etc., and then going to Jewish balls and weddings."[82] Spivak's involvement in so many aspects of Philadelphia's Jewish society—both formal and informal—which Ball alludes to, is confirmed by a letter Spivak wrote on February 27, 1896. The letter, handwritten on stationery that bears the imprint, "Dr. C.D. Spivak, 529 Pine Street," is addressed to the president of the Jewish Orphan Guardians Society and reads: "On account of sickness in my family I am compelled to leave the city shortly for Denver Colorado, and it will be impossible for me to attend the meeting tonight. For the same reason I respectfully tender herewith my resignation as guardian."[83]

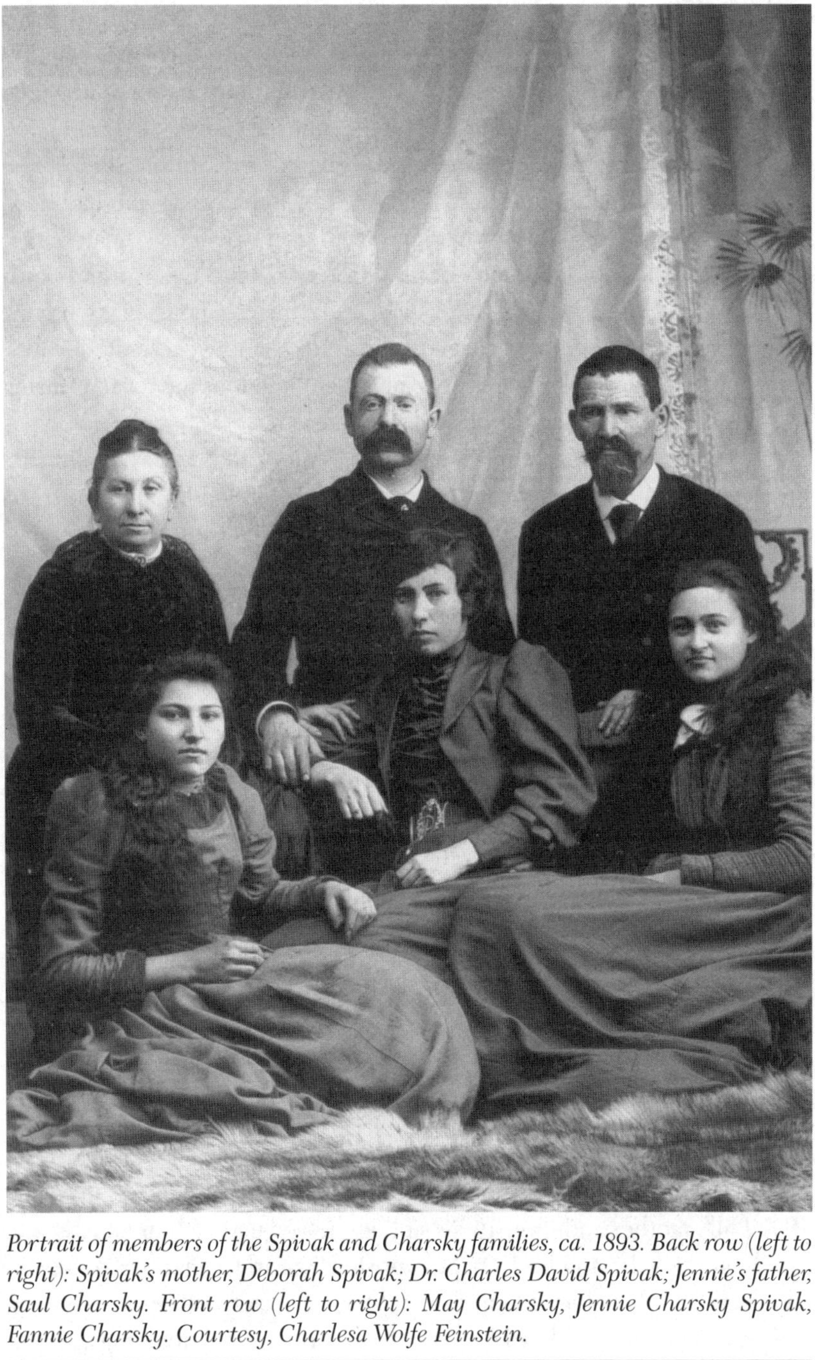

Portrait of members of the Spivak and Charsky families, ca. 1893. Back row (left to right): Spivak's mother, Deborah Spivak; Dr. Charles David Spivak; Jennie's father, Saul Charsky. Front row (left to right): May Charsky, Jennie Charsky Spivak, Fannie Charsky. Courtesy, Charlesa Wolfe Feinstein.

The next night nearly fifty friends sponsored a surprise goodbye party for Jennie and Charles Spivak to wish them luck with their move and in their new home in the American West. The group was made up of Philadelphia's Russian immigrant Jewish intellectual community, including fellow physicians and students. Among the guests were Simon Skidelsky, a Philadelphia journalist, and his wife, Dr. Rachel Skidelsky, who had been a colleague of Spivak's at the Maimonides Clinic dispensary; theater critic David Apotheker; photographer Elias Goldensky; and the Spivak boarders, Abraham Margolin and Dr. Leo Noy Gartman, among many others. The repast assembled by the guests included sandwiches, pfeffernuss, tarts, wine, beer, whiskey, and especially the ubiquitous Samovar, offering the tea so popular with Russian Jewish immigrants.[84]

Michael Ball was also present at the party and had his own comments on the evening, as well as about the departure of his longtime friends. His recollections were recorded several months after the events:

> Spivak's going was bound up with a few incidents. We, that is, some of his near friends, gave him a surprise party, at which I was initiated as a Russian. It was a jolly crowd and much was made of the fact that it was a surprise. Then we gave him a little dinner at Boothby's. Afterwards, I went to live at Spivak's house. . . . Gradually the time came for their departure. We were a large crowd at the Depot, and then good-bye. I returned, took possession of the house, my furniture had arrived, and in a few days, the other party, who were to be my tenants, came with their things.[85]

It took Dr. Ball some time to settle into Spivak's practice. He noted, "My practice in the first month was fairly good," but "[t]he second and third months of my work were not as good as the first month, and the fourth month has been dull, but the bad times are again upon us, and no one has work. I think I have lost a number of Spivak's patients, but I have others in their place. I am again discouraged because I do not make expenses." He complained that "[t]he Russian homes are extremely filthy, but the people are fond of their children and fairly hospitable."[86] In spring 1897 Ball's mother and three of his siblings moved in with him for a time to "keep house."[87] In August 1897 he reported, "Nearly a year has gone, and what have I to show for it? I am still at 529 Pine Street, still working among the poor Russian Jews, but I have more of a home. After debating one way and another, after wondering whether Spivak would return or no, parents and I decided to stay here."[88]

Dr. Charles Spivak did not return to resume his practice in Philadelphia. By the 1890s Colorado had achieved a national reputation as the "World's Sanatorium," and the Spivaks had joined thousands of others to "chase the cure" in Denver, the state's Queen City. Jennie Spivak probably suffered from incipient tuberculosis, although family legend suggested she merely had bronchitis. It seems this would have been an unlikely reason for Charles Spivak to have uprooted his family and given up his growing practice in Philadelphia. More likely, Dr. Spivak, who was devoted to his wife, felt that given the contemporary medical belief that a dry, sunny climate and high altitude afforded the best chance for a cure for consumption—the most dreaded disease of the era—Colorado offered a good opportunity for recovery. The move was indeed fateful, one that would set Spivak on his future mission as a crusader for an innovative, compassionate, and culturally sensitive treatment of tuberculosis—the leading cause of death in America when the Spivaks settled in Denver in 1896.

Although in Philadelphia Spivak had been known as a leading gastroenterologist, in Denver he would also build his reputation as a leader in the field of tuberculosis treatment, and his name would become well-known around the United States as the guiding genius of the Jewish Consumptives' Relief Society. In a memorial published in *The American Review of Tuberculosis* in 1927, two months after Spivak's death, his eulogizer concluded: "In the passing of Doctor Spivak the sanatorium movement has lost one of its pioneer and valiant workers. . . . Side by side with the research worker in the anti-tuberculosis movement is the promoter and builder of institutions to harbor the sufferers from the White Plague. . . . When the history of the campaign against this dread disease is written due credit will surely be given to the organizer and sanatorium builder—Charles David Spivak."[89]

4

Heading West to "Chase the Cure"

Today, most people in the United States consider tuberculosis a disease of the past and view it with clinical detachment. Others may be vaguely aware that tuberculosis still affects a number of U.S. citizens, mainly those who are impoverished, elderly, or have compromised immune systems. It also continues to pose a considerable threat in underdeveloped countries. Yet at the end of the nineteenth century tuberculosis, or consumption and the "White Plague," as the disease was also commonly known, was the leading cause of death in the United States. The word "tuberculosis" alone was enough to invoke fear in the hearts of countless Americans. Dr. Edward Trudeau, the generally acknowledged founder of the sanatorium movement in America and himself a victim of tuberculosis, vividly recalled his reaction to being diagnosed with the disease. "I think I know something of the feeling of the man at the bar who is told he is to be hanged on a given date," he wrote, "for in those days, pulmonary consumption was considered absolutely fatal. . . . I was stunned."[1]

When Charles and Jennie Spivak arrived in Denver in 1896 in search of a more healthful climate for Jennie, the city was still suffering from the effects of the economic depression of 1893. The gold that had initially helped launch Denver aided in the city's recovery as well when the Cripple Creek gold bonanza began in the 1890s. By 1900 Denver's population had grown to 133,859, and impressive mansions and landmarks such as the famous Brown Palace Hotel dotted the landscape. At the same time, a booming health "industry" was attracting hundreds and later thousands of men and women to Denver and Colorado Springs to "chase the cure" and seek a remedy for tuberculosis, the most dreaded disease of the era. Many of the health seekers who traveled to Colorado to take advantage of its climate died; others recovered and returned to their former homes. A significant number, however, like the Spivaks, settled in Colorado to begin a new life. Although the exact number is subject to debate, by the 1920s as much as 60 percent of Colorado's population may have migrated to the state—either directly or indirectly—for treatment of tuberculosis.[2] These new migrants substantially affected Colorado's social, economic, and political development, not just its medical history. Dr. Charles David Spivak was one of those who left an indelible mark.

Although tuberculosis was an ancient disease, with evidence of its occurrence at least as far back as early Egyptian times, progress in its control and eradication was virtually nonexistent for centuries.[3] Prior to bacteriologist Robert Koch's discovery of the tubercle bacillus in 1882, most physicians felt tuberculosis was a hereditary and non-communicable disease best treated in a favorable climate supplemented by long-term exposure to fresh air and a proper diet.[4] Even Trudeau, the "father" of the American sanatorium movement, seemed unaware at first that tuberculosis was contagious. In the 1860s he nursed his consumptive brother without taking any special precautions. The close contact with his sick brother was probably the source of Trudeau's own tuberculosis.[5] Today, tuberculosis is understood as an infectious disease caused by the tubercle bacillus, a rod-shaped bacterium germ. Tuberculosis can affect many body organs, including the brain, liver, and kidneys, but the most common form—pulmonary tuberculosis—is generally spread from person to person through the air by droplets from an infected individual with an active case of the disease who has coughed or sneezed. Most of these droplets prove harmless, but sometimes residue droplet nuclei settle in the lungs of another susceptible host and cause a new infection.[6]

Open-air therapy for pulmonary tuberculosis, which became a cornerstone of American sanatorium treatment, had long been utilized in Colorado.[7] No single accepted standard for tuberculosis treatment prevailed in the early years, but by 1880 medical opinion emphasized fresh air for respiratory ailments. Colorado, with its dry, sunny climate, drew tuberculosis victims like a magnet. Certainly, the ultraviolet rays in Colorado's abundant sunshine proved a valuable tool in preventing the spread of the disease outdoors. In 1887 the Denver Chamber of Commerce proudly proclaimed Colorado "the mecca for consumptives, and rightfully; for dry air, equitable temperature, and continuous sunshine are as yet the most reliable factors in the care of that disease." The report went on to boast that tuberculosis "is generally cured and always benefited by permanent residence here."[8]

As early as 1859, the year of the Pikes Peak gold rush and the first wave of Anglo settlers into the area, local boosters were already singing the region's praises. Over the next half century physicians, railroad and city promoters, and journalists, among others, became converts to the health-giving properties of the Rocky Mountains. In a booklet titled *The Heart of the Rockies*, for example, published by the Denver & Rio Grande Railroad in 1880, the author maintained that "the invalid of the east, with hollow eyes and shrunken faces," could find a cure for his or her illness in the areas' "salubrious and health giving climate."[9]

It is not surprising, then, that long before Denver medical-based sanatoriums appeared around the turn of the twentieth century, tuberculosis victims had employed informal and sometimes ingenious methods to maximize their exposure to the supposed benefits of Colorado's high altitude and invigorating dry, fresh air. Apparently heeding one early Colorado physician's advice that "tubercular cases cannot expect to get well unless they come here determined to live out-of-doors in the sunshine, and in the fresh air,"[10] many consumptives braved all sorts of weather. This appears to have been a common practice, for as Thomas Galbreath observed during his stay in Colorado: "It is not unusual to see an invalid sitting on a covered porch, overcoated, furred, and blanketed with hot bricks or a hot-water bag at his feet, while snow is swirling and drifting over him, and the thermometer not above zero. At night, he sleeps on a porch, in a tent, or in a room with every window open, and when he reaches for the glass of water by his bedside, he is frequently denied the drink he wants, because it is frozen hard."[11]

Denver in particular became known nationally as a center of hope for tuberculosis victims, who learned of its beneficial climate though medical and popular publications, by word of mouth, or from concerted booster efforts.[12] Historian Billy Jones has pointed out that "no portion of the health frontier with the possible exception of Southern California, received greater nationwide publicity after the Civil War than Colorado."[13] Paradoxically, while Denver boosters actively wooed consumptives in the early years, little thought was given to providing proper facilities for those who required more than a little "invigorating air." Even before the turn of the century, this problem had become acute. Consumptives who had flocked to Denver in the hope of finding a cure were often unable to secure simple lodging, let alone medical care.

As germ theory and the communicable nature of the disease became better understood, the state that for many years had courted consumptives to raise its capital and increase its population soon shunned them. The new science of bacteriology increasingly emphasized that the disease could be spread through "indiscriminate" coughing and sneezing and warned against contact with tuberculosis victims. Thus Thomas Galbreath, a young easterner who had come to Colorado at the turn of the century because of his poor health, found the city decidedly inhospitable. "Colorado," he declared bitterly, "is most glad to welcome the contents of the purse the invalid brings with him, but she would greatly prefer that the invalid should not accompany the purse."[14]

For the most part, state and municipal authorities abrogated responsibility for the victims of the White Plague, and it was left to private parties, such as concerned individuals and local ethnic and religious groups, to remedy the increasingly critical public health situation. Charles Spivak probably supervised his wife Jennie's medical regimen himself, or the dry climate and high altitude might have simply worked their reputed magic on her as they did for many others who were not too seriously ill when they arrived. Their daughter Deena Spivak Strauss recalled that the Spivak family first found temporary quarters in a boardinghouse that catered to tuberculosis victims run by a teacher named Mrs. Edgerton, who later became an early supporter of the Jewish Consumptives' Relief Society.[15]

Dr. Charles Spivak was also part of a significant migration of physicians to Colorado. During the late nineteenth century, Colorado attracted many doctors who came not only to establish their practices and secure a better income but often also for their own health or that of family members. In a 1908 essay in the *Denver Medical Times*, Dr. A. C. Magruder reported that 32.7 percent of the state's physicians had come to Colorado because they or someone in their family suffered from tuberculosis.[16] Not surprisingly, many like Dr. Spivak eventually made tuberculosis their specialty. This was certainly the case with Dr. Charles Denison, who became perhaps the most ardent supporter of Colorado's climate and one of its most effective boosters. He arrived in Colorado in 1873 to seek a cure, and his book, *Rocky Mountain Health Resorts*, probably did more than any other single publication to attract consumptives to the state.[17] For years Denison extolled the virtues of altitude, and as late as 1908 he was still making his views known in essays such as "How Does Climate Influence Tuberculosis?"[18]

Denison, an acknowledged tuberculosis specialist, was only one of many physicians who argued for the benefits of Colorado's climate. Leading medical journals such as the *Denver Medical Times*, *Colorado Climatologist*, and *Colorado Medical Journal* in the 1880s, 1890s, and the first decade of the twentieth century also carried articles on the subject. Although there were some dissenters, most Colorado doctors regarded the state's climate as inherently hostile to tuberculosis. Even when the benefit of climate was seriously debated and Koch's discovery of the communicability of tuberculosis was widely accepted, Colorado physicians such as Luther Woods were still claiming great local advantages. "Few facts," he stated," are better attested than . . . the benefits to be derived from the Colorado climate by the consumptive."[19]

Outside Colorado, however, physicians promoting local treatment disagreed with physicians such as Woods. Dr. Lawrence Flick of Philadelphia, for example, who became one of the leaders of the national tuberculosis crusade, maintained in contrast that it "is much better that a consumptive have home comforts in the worst climate in the world than that he be compelled to undergo the tortures of boardinghouse or fourth-class hotel at a health resort."[20] However, Flick was not referring to the formal medical sanatoriums that sprang up in Colorado after the turn of the century. In any case, numerous seriously ill consumptives often pursued a last chance in Colorado's famed environment in their desperate search for a cure, despite medical advice that discouraged such endeavors.

Like other states in the West, such as California, Arizona, and New Mexico, Colorado had advertised the advantages of local climate for health seekers, hoping to attract new settlers who would increase business in the state. This campaign resulted in several unanticipated results. As Galbreath perceptively summed up the situation in another book he wrote on the life of tuberculosis victims, "Colorado as a resort country has been so fancifully written up time and again, that it is small wonder that invalids come here, *sans* money, *sans* friends, *sans* sufficient clothes even, expecting that, in some miraculous way, money and clothes and friends and health will all descend upon them while they sleep."[21] Moreover, wide advertising attracted not only those who might make a financial contribution to the growth of the state but also many more "who brought nothing except their hope for cure," resulting in the development of a public health crisis of major proportions.[22] As more indigent tuberculosis victims arrived, Denver was faced with what a contemporary social worker called "one of the most complex social phenomenon of our day."[23]

Despite the growing challenge, assistance for the tide of tuberculosis victims was slow in coming. Before the opening of National Jewish Hospital for Consumptives in 1899, beds for consumptive patients in city and state general hospital facilities were so scarce that the poor were frequently left to their own devices, sometimes dying in the streets. While affluent tuberculosis victims were often able to find a boardinghouse, hotel, or an exclusive sanatorium like Cragmor in Colorado Springs, the prospects for consumptive men and women who were doubly afflicted with disease and poverty were bleak. As the years progressed, injunctions to keep poor consumptives out of Colorado became more overt. In 1908 Dr. Sherman Bonney, a well-known Colorado tuberculosis specialist, wrote, "There can be no greater error than sending the hopeless, indigent patient to health resorts."[24]

Of course, the stigma attached to poor consumptives was not only a Colorado phenomenon, and the disease nationally came to reflect a social as well as a medical component that frequently equated tuberculosis in a negative manner with the lower working classes, especially immigrants. Indeed, after 1900 tuberculosis *was* most prevalent among the low-income population, particularly immigrants and people of color.[25] Individuals with compromised immune systems as a result of poor nutrition, overwork, and unhealthy living and working conditions were understandably the most susceptible to the disease. But many blamed the poor's "bad habits" for their illness rather than inequitable social conditions or circumstances beyond their control. In other words, the upper and middle classes often viewed the poor as agents of the disease rather than victims and as a menacing threat to public health.[26] Dr. Flick treated both the rich and poor in Philadelphia, but it was the impoverished tuberculosis victims who claimed his greatest sympathy and whom he observed experienced the greatest challenge, as their condition was generally met with "indifference, fear or loathing."[27]

In Colorado, several factors contributed to the indifference toward consumptives. First, the increasing fear of contracting the disease made many people reluctant to have any direct contact with tuberculars. Second, the celebrated emphasis on individualism associated with the West presented drawbacks in dealing with public health issues, as emphasis on self-reliance tended to shift responsibility away from the community at large. As historian Michael Teller has pointed out, in this regard it is logical that historically, for the most part, northeastern and midwestern states generally took the initiative in public health and social welfare.[28] In addition, as Gunther Barth has noted, Denver developed as an "instant city" that "raced through the entire process of American city building, crowding a century into one generation." Focused on the race for profit, many Denver citizens "showed a remarkable indifference to most aspects of urban life that did not directly affect their pursuit of wealth."[29]

As state government and city leaders continued to pretend the tuberculosis problem did not exist, in Denver four voluntary religio-ethnic sanatoriums initiated the first concerted effort to deal with the growing plight of destitute or struggling consumptives: National Jewish Hospital (NJH), which opened in 1899; the Jewish Consumptives' Relief Society (JCRS), which followed in 1904; the Evangelical Lutheran Sanatorium, which opened in 1905; and the Swedish National Sanatorium, which was incorporated in 1905 and began providing services in 1908. While immigrants in urban centers across the nation were never totally isolated from one another, most of these newcomers tended to cluster in their own ethnic neighborhood enclaves. This general pattern spilled over into the founding of Denver's religio-ethnic based hospitals as well. In organizing their health care institutions as sanatoriums, these four hospitals were also taking a prominent role in the larger medical movement sweeping the country around 1900. In 1884 Dr. Edward Trudeau opened his pathbreaking sanatorium in the Adirondack Mountains at Saranac Lake in upstate

New York, and similar institutions soon dotted the American landscape. The common therapy provided in most sanatoriums, which included a regimen of nutritious food, adequate rest, and maximum exposure to fresh air—all under close medical supervision—was beyond the means of those with limited incomes. For the most part, only philanthropy or public funds could help those tuberculosis patients unable to give up their jobs for a sustained period of rest or to pay for the associated medical services.

In fact, it was the tiny Jewish community in Denver in the late nineteenth century that made the first organized efforts to come to the aid of impoverished tuberculosis victims who were pouring into the state. The Jewish population in Colorado was only about 1,500 in 1897, the year after Jennie and Charles settled in the Mile High City,[30] but as early as the 1880s a prominent local Jewish woman of German descent, Frances Wisebart Jacobs, had made destitute consumptives her personal cause. Frances had arrived in Central City, Colorado, in 1863 as the young bride of clothing merchant Abraham Jacobs, who was active in local politics.[31] When the family moved to Denver, Frances, who later earned the sobriquet "Denver's Mother of Charities," moved within a proper "women's sphere" at the time, caring for the ill and impoverished. A bright, forceful, and energetic woman, Jacobs was typical of many middle-class women of her generation, who channeled their talents into what was regarded as a suitable and respectable role for a woman—that of nurturer and healer.[32] In addition to being the primary impetus behind the creation of NJH, in 1887 Mrs. Jacobs, along with a Catholic priest and a Protestant minister, organized the Denver Charity Organization Society (COS)—a federation of charities that was the forerunner of the Community Chest, which, in turn, evolved into the modern national United Way. She also introduced the first free kindergarten to Denver.[33]

Frances Jacobs pursued a relentless campaign to provide care for indigent tuberculosis victims, but her entreaties were initially rebuffed because local leaders feared bad publicity for the city and state that might blacken their image as a health resort. Jacobs was, however, able to use her considerable persuasive talents to enlist the interest of the local Jewish population, later led by Rabbi William Friedman of Denver's Reform temple, Congregation Emanuel, who also became a driving force in the creation of National Jewish Hospital. The result was the Jewish Hospital Association, incorporated in 1890, which collected funds for a building at the corner of Colfax Avenue and Colorado Boulevard. Unfortunately, Frances Jacobs died before the hospital opened, but initially it was named the Frances Jacobs Hospital in her memory. Because of financial problems, the hospital stood empty for many years and did not open until 1899, when B'nai B'rith, a national Jewish fraternal organization, came to its rescue.[34] In recognition of this national support, the hospital opened under a new name, the National Jewish Hospital for Consumptives, and with its opening the sanatorium movement had arrived in Denver. The institution was unique in that it was the first in the state and probably the entire country to make the free treatment of indigent victims its primary goal, operating under the motto "None May Enter Who Can Pay—None Can Pay Who Enter."

When Charles and Jennie Spivak arrived at Denver's Union Station in 1896 with their small son David and baby daughter Deena, the depot, including its distinctive clock tower, had been newly renovated following a damaging fire that occurred in 1894. Characterized by historians as an "instant" city, between 1870 and 1900 Denver's population grew from 4,749 to 133,859, and railroads had been a central factor in the city's transformation from a mining camp to a bustling metropolis. One hundred trains arrived and departed daily from Union Station, the gateway to the Mile High City. Within the city itself, in addition to horse-drawn wagons, buggies, and carriages, a network of streetcars transported Denver's citizens from one neighborhood to another.

Charles Spivak entered the story of tuberculosis treatment in Colorado almost from his arrival in 1896, when the Frances Jacobs Hospital building was standing but dormant as it awaited the necessary cash infusion to open its doors. Spivak's interest in the prevention and treatment of the disease was probably sparked during his early practice in Philadelphia. He may have personally known Dr. Lawrence Flick, who had helped organize the Pennsylvania Society for the Prevention of Tuberculosis in that city in 1892 and served as the organization's first president. Flick's Free Hospital for Poor Consumptives, which opened in Philadelphia in 1895, may also have influenced Spivak's views on what he considered proper care for indigent tuberculosis patients.

Spivak's concern about tuberculosis care in Denver is evidenced by a series of letters written in June and July 1897 on the stationery of the Denver and Arapahoe Medical Society, of which he was secretary. The address of his first medical office appears on the letterhead as 608 California Building in downtown Denver. In these letters, Spivak discussed various suggestions for obtaining funding to open NJH. He strongly advocated turning the "Denver Jewish Hospital" into a national organization and initially hoped to enlist the assistance of the National Council of Jewish Women (NCJW).[35] The NCJW had been created in 1893 as an outgrowth of the Congress of Jewish Women at the Chicago World's Columbian Exposition. Two of its early goals were to increase knowledge among American Jewish women and encourage philanthropy and social reform. A Denver "section," or chapter, was initiated in 1893 with Carrie Benjamin as president.[36]

At Spivak's urging, Denver NCJW chapter representatives made an attempt to "induce the National Council of Jewish Women and through it the Jewish women of the whole land to open and maintain the Jewish hospital in Denver under its auspices." Dr. Spivak then undertook a public relations campaign aimed at influential Jewish periodicals. In a letter to the Philadelphia *Jewish Exponent,* he outlined the history of the "Jewish Hospital in the city [Denver], whose doors were never opened to receive patients. . . . I have evolved in my mind various schemes and plans how to open the hospital and save it from falling into ruin, but none were satisfactory." Spivak concluded that the plan was now in the hands of those who could carry it through, and he invited the newspaper's public support.[37]

Although the details are unclear, the NCJW did not come to the aid of the hospital, but salvation eventually came through the national B'nai B'rith organization, which helped underwrite the opening of the formally non-sectarian National Jewish Hospital in 1899 through a head tax on individual members nationally. NJH operated as a sanatorium for tuberculosis patients, with the typical emphasis on fresh air, rest, and diet. The word "hospital" was used in its title, however, to convey that patients would receive medical care from a trained staff of doctors and nurses rather than being in an informal camp-like setting that characterized many similar early undertakings. While the first patient to enter the NJH was a young gentile Swedish woman,[38] according to the NJH's *First Annual Report*, 82 of the first 149 patients at the sanatorium were East European Jewish immigrants,[39] a pattern that continued at least until the 1930s.

By the time Spivak was agitating for the opening of the first national Jewish tuberculosis sanatorium, he was already well-known in Denver.

Shortly after Charles and Jennie arrived, he became active in the Denver medical community as a popular clinician and soon gained the respect of his peers. The Spivaks settled in a middle-class neighborhood at the edge of Denver's downtown area rather than in the Jewish immigrant East European West Colfax enclave, probably reflecting their upwardly mobile middle-class status and a desire for Spivak's medical practice to be more centrally located. According to Deena Spivak Strauss, the family's first home in Denver was a terrace apartment near 12th Street and Welton, near what became the Emily Griffith Opportunity School. However, an interesting situation that arose soon after Spivak's arrival in Denver is illustrative of his continuing commitment to fellow East European immigrants and his efforts to nurture budding physicians. When a young immigrant Jewish medical student from the Midwest with whom Spivak had corresponded wrote to say he was unable to complete his medical studies because of strained financial circumstances, Spivak immediately responded, "[d]on't drop [your] studies. Come to Denver, live with us to make your living expenses small. I'll adjust your tuition fee to a very small amount."[40]

The young man, the future Dr. M. Sahud of Chicago, joined the Spivak family in their modest residence for his last year at the University of Denver's Department of Medicine, where Spivak was one of his instructors. Sahud offers a unique insider's perspective of the core personality behind Spivak's public persona, which according to the student were one and the same:

> The cordiality and simplicity of both of them [Charles and Jennie] left no room for the embarrassment I thought I would feel as a new comer. . . . Now I had the opportunity to study Dr. Spivak at close range—at home, at work, as a teacher, and as a social worker. His life was an open one. . . . His face, his smile, his quiet walk, the fire in his calm speech, when he privately or publicly expressed his ideas, were always the same. Spivak at home, on the platform, in his office with patients, or [later] in the JCRS Sanatorium, was always the embodiment of sympathy, justice, and good sense.[41]

Considering the struggles Spivak had faced in his early life—particularly during his turbulent student days in Russia and Philadelphia, as a recent immigrant struggling to make a living, and then as a newly minted physician—he must have made a conscious and concerted effort to develop that calm demeanor.

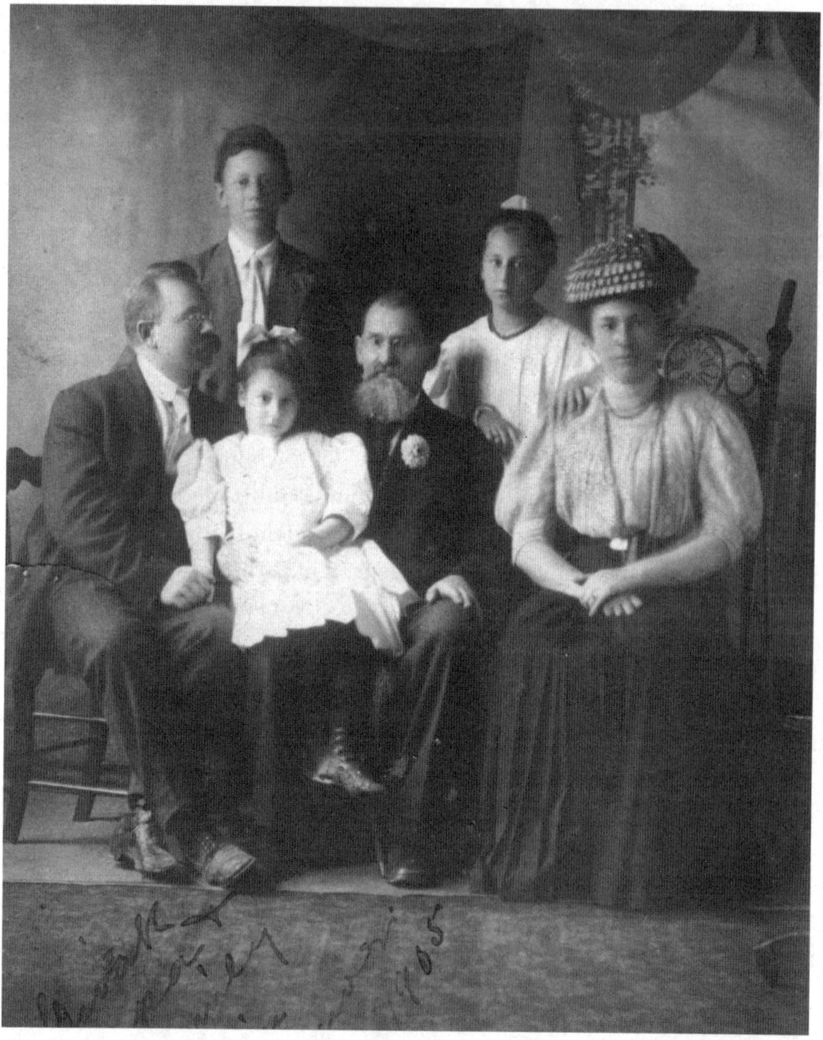

The Spivak family in 1905. Standing (left to right): David Spivak, Deena Spivak. Seated (left to right): Dr. Charles David Spivak, Ruth Spivak, Saul Charsky, Jennie Charsky Spivak. Courtesy, Charlesa Wolfe Feinstein.

Even though Spivak became a prominent Denver resident, he retained lifelong friendships with people across the country. Spivak was an inveterate letter writer, and his correspondence is filled with charm and vivid descriptions. One of his most valued correspondents was Judge

Mayer Sulzberger, the noted Philadelphia Jewish jurist, to whom Spivak often turned for advice. Sulzberger had encouraged him to take up a project that resulted in a lengthy article titled "Medicine in the Bible and the Talmud," which was published in the *Jewish Encyclopedia* in 1901. In a letter he wrote to Sulzberger in 1904 from Denver, Spivak alluded to his strong passion for writing and confessed that he sometimes suffered from "an acute exacerbation of 'writer's itch.'"[42] One of Spivak's most useful talents was his ability to write for both a professional and a popular audience with equal ease.

From 1896 to 1901, Dr. Charles Spivak served as an associate professor in the Department of Medicine at the University of Denver and as a professor of anatomy in 1897–1898, as well as assuming the chair of gastroenterology.[43] He may have been the first Jewish faculty member in the medical school. According to Sahud, Spivak took over the anatomy class on short notice, preparing in only three months during the summer. Still, Sahud observed that "from the very first lecture [Spivak was able] to bewitch the students, and become the most popular professor. The dead bones, muscles, nerves, and blood vessels took on new life in his lectures, began again to perform their functions."[44]

As Sahud had observed, Spivak's animated personality and engaging manner of lecturing made him an admired teacher, and his Denver students published an outline of his lectures in 1900, the year Spivak became a professor of clinical medicine at the Denver and Gross College of Medicine. He served in that position until 1907. A medical colleague recalled that "Dr. Spivak's lectures were well attended because of the manner in which they were delivered. Even his lectures on anatomy were not dry. They were presented in a literary style, and showed the relationship of anatomy to clinical medicine and to everyday life."[45] During this period Spivak was elected secretary of the Denver and Arapahoe Medical College in 1897 and president of the Colorado Medical Society in 1902.[46]

In the field of gastroenterology, Spivak developed a significant reputation, both locally in his private practice and through scientific articles published in distinguished medical journals. In 1898 Spivak published his first article in the *Journal of the American Medical Association* (JAMA), the nation's most prestigious medical publication. His essay, "Rest—A Neglected Factor in the Treatment of Gastro Intestinal Disorder," brought his then novel approach to treating stomach problems to national attention. He subsequently published many articles on the subject. Spivak emphasized a conservative approach of bed rest, a controlled diet, and hot poultices at a time when most physicians relied on invasive stomach washes, painful techniques, and drugs to treat intestinal disease. Spivak wrote: "I wish to raise my voice many octaves above a whisper, and proclaim loudly and boldly that I employ rest, nature's greatest panacea, as my first and best weapon against the greatest foe of mankind—diseases of the gastrointestinal tract. I know that the tendency of our time is to treat diseases of the stomach by washing, scouring, scratching, punching, and electrifying the stomach."[47] Spivak's reliance on rest in the treatment of stomach disease also later became a major weapon in his battle against tuberculosis.

Spivak's lively writing style is evident even in his medical publications. As English was not his native tongue, his writing facility in that language was impressive. Spivak's first foray into formal medical literature had occurred shortly after he graduated from Philadelphia's Jefferson Medical College, when his prize-winning essay on menstruation was published in *The Times and Register*. While his medical writings focused primarily on subjects relating to gastroenterology, his scope was wide-ranging. In 1896, for example, he published an essay titled "Delivery at Term after Ten Previous Consecutive Abortions" in *The American Gynecological and Obstetrical Journal*. Many have noted Spivak's ability to take dry subjects and make them appealing. His wit is evident both in his style and in the provocative titles he chose, such as one article on gastroenterology called "The Whistle in the Stomach. Who Blew It First? A Question of Priority," which appeared in the normally staid JAMA in 1905.[48]

Spivak also used his research and writing to merge his Jewish and medical interests. He was especially fond of what would be termed medical history, particularly when it related to Jewish themes in the Bible and the Talmud. In addition to his well-known essay in *The Jewish Encyclopedia*, Spivak published several articles on Jewish customs as they related to medical practice as well as an unusual but intriguing piece on the topic of general literature called "Physicians in Fiction: Physicians as Seen by Henry Fielding," in a 1905 issue of the *Journal of the American Medical Association*. This was one of several articles in a series that examined medical characters in works by such prominent European writers as Shakespeare and Moliere.[49]

Spivak was an astonishingly prolific writer. A bibliography of his known writings published in *Medical Life* in 1928, a year after his death, listed 150 publications. They included works on medical history, medical bibliography, technical medical writings, and numerous articles aimed at a popular audience, including many in English but some in Yiddish, Hebrew, and Russian as well.[50] Once Spivak became associated with the JCRS, he often traveled long distances by train on behalf of the sanatorium. Perhaps these trips provided the opportunity to compose drafts. Certainly, his files contain many notes for articles and speeches written on stationery from hotels all over the United States. Over the years his medical pieces appeared in a variety of well-established publications such as *Journal of the American Medical Association*, *Medical Record*, *Medical Times*, *The Colorado Medical Journal*, *The New York Medical Journal*, and *American Medicine*, while his general compositions were featured in many newspapers across the country.

As his early colleague and friend Dr. Michael Ball had observed, the ebullient Spivak was always full of schemes and plans, some of which never came to fruition. However, one of his earliest successes in Denver resulted from his concern that published medical knowledge be disseminated to local physicians who often had little access to major medical libraries. Spivak's creative solution to the problem was the introduction of his ambitious Union Catalogue Plan to the Denver and Arapahoe Medical Society.

In discussing the Union Catalogue in an 1897 issue of *The Colorado Medical Journal*, Spivak noted the proliferation of medical literature and the fact that many local doctors sometimes received unsolicited and unwanted reprints of journal articles that fell outside their personal interests as gifts from fellow physicians who had authored an essay. Spivak's novel approach was to pool the varied medical works scattered in the libraries of individual doctors in Denver that were not available in the public medical library, catalog them, and make the material available to all local physicians who would then be able to consult or borrow from one another once they were apprised of the location and ownership of the material they sought. A master list would be deposited at the Denver Medical Society library.[51] Spivak's project was later praised by the head librarian at the Denver Public Library: "Dr. C. D. Spivak suggested the idea of a union catalogue of medical libraries of Denver physicians. He was appointed a committee to carry out this idea. He performed his task so well that the catalogue was completed before the middle of the year."[52]

The Union Catalogue Plan also earned the Denver physician a national reputation. The project was noted with great appreciation in JAMA: "Dr. Spivak has himself suggested an important idea and has carried it into practical effect in connection with the Colorado Medical Society of Denver. . . . In this way he was able to add more than 6,000 volumes to the medical works generally available for reference to the profession in Denver." Moreover, the journal recommended that "[s]ome such plan might be followed in any large town or city, and would be of very wide benefit to the profession."[53] Spivak thus became known nationally as somewhat of an expert on medical literature by the end of the nineteenth century. In fact, in 1902 an article by Spivak titled "Medical Reprints" was published in JAMA.[54]

The level of respect Spivak received from Colorado's early medical community is also evident in the fact that he was immediately suggested to head another new project. From 1898 to 1902, Dr. Charles Spivak served as the editor of a monthly periodical in Denver called *Medical Libraries*, an outgrowth of the earlier *Monthly Bulletin* of the Colorado Medical Library Association. Under Spivak's direction, the primary aims of the new publication were to encourage the founding of medical collections in public libraries, the compilation of union catalogs of medical publications around the country, and the organization of a national Medical Library Association—Spivak's pet project. By May 1898 Spivak happily reported that the latter had come into existence following a meeting in Philadelphia.[55]

By 1899, the publication's second year, Spivak could boast that "we are happy to say that our subscription list is made up of men who are the leaders of the medical profession in the United States." Subscribers included Dr. William Osler, a professor at Johns Hopkins Medical School in Baltimore, who was one of the most famous physicians in the country and who specialized in tuberculosis treatment. In the same issue, Spivak authored an important article on "The Medical Libraries of the United States," which not only detailed the existence of these institutions but also provided insight into his own medical philosophy, which emphasized his lifelong commitment to education as an ongoing process. "Every conscientious physician," he wrote, "even from the best equipped medical schools, will acknowledge that the three or four years of collegiate study were simply years of preparation. Real knowledge of the science and art of medicine is post-graduate, and is acquired slowly and gradually. The longer one is in practice the more this fact impresses itself upon the mind. Life is one long post-graduate course, which we take in different ways, in different institutions, and from different teachers."[56]

Spivak's welcoming reception within the general Denver community at the turn of the twentieth century reflected the wide acceptance of Jewish citizens in the early American West. Despite their distinction as a religious minority, pioneer Jews in communities throughout the region were generally viewed as a stabilizing influence that upheld morality and order in new settlements and brought a measure of culture to the rough frontier. Because society in the early frontier West was relatively fluid, with a more open and pragmatic class and social structure, Jews appear to have been accorded more power and opportunity than their counterparts in other areas of the United States, and they were frequently welcomed as partners in building a new social order. Historian Earl Pomeroy has observed that "newcomers were especially welcome in the nineteenth-century West, above all in villages and towns ambitious to become cities."[57] Jewish merchants initially helped build Denver, and "where immigrants established themselves economically, they also established themselves politically."[58]

Moreover, recent studies of religion in the American West have argued that because the region never produced a single religious mainstream, relatively significant mutual tolerance was present, and "in most areas the three historic faiths—Protestantism, Catholicism, Judaism—coexisted with relative equanimity."[59] Charles Spivak certainly benefited from the respected and pivotal role early Jewish residents had played in Denver's growth and development as he, in turn, developed his own local reputation. Even as Spivak successfully mingled with and worked among leading members of Denver's general community, he demonstrated a strong sense of Jewish identity. It is especially ironic that, as we shall see later, Spivak was more challenged by intra-ethnic tensions than by members of other ethnic and religious groups he encountered in Colorado's Queen City of the Plains.

In the meantime, as her husband became more prominent, Jennie Spivak was establishing her own intellectual and artistic niche in the Denver community. When Jennie stepped off the train in 1896 to make

Denver her new home, women in Denver were already exercising their right to cast a ballot—a watershed event in expanding women's rights that must have greatly pleased the progressive Jennie, for she was certainly an advocate of female suffrage. In 1893, women's suffrage was approved by popular male vote through a state referendum in Colorado, making Denver the largest city in the United States at the time in which women could vote.[60]

After delays in Philadelphia, in 1904 Jennie completed her college degree at the University of Denver and joined the school's faculty as an instructor of Russian from 1903 to 1913.[61] Sharing her husband's gift for languages, Jennie spoke fluent German and French as well as English. Apparently proud of her university position, the independent-minded Jennie maintained a separate listing from her husband in the *Denver City Directory*, which over the years variously named her as professor or teacher. By that time both Charles and Jennie listed their downtown address as 1421 Court Place, which served as both Spivak's office and their place of residence. Sometime in 1907 the family moved to a fine new brick home in a sedate middle-class neighborhood much closer to the University of Denver at 850 South Franklin, which overlooked the lake at Washington Park, one of Denver's most beautiful landmarks. Jennie also became active in the JCRS and involved as a prominent member of Denver's elite Why Club, a women's literary and discussion group, while she was teaching and raising a family. She was later honored for her work in education when she was named a "Representative Woman of Colorado."[62]

It is puzzling that, given Spivak's prominence in Denver and his active role in promoting the cause of opening National Jewish Hospital, he ultimately did not become involved in its beginning operations and development. Some clues to the mystery emerge from an examination of the antagonisms present at the turn of the twentieth century between the established German Jewish community and the East European immigrants, which involved significant differences in contemporary medical opinion on the best course of treatment for tuberculosis patients as well as individual local rivalries. To better understand the situation, we first need to briefly examine the early history of NJH.

Jewish tradition, which placed great emphasis on responsibility for the sick and indigent, influenced the Denver Jewish community's pivotal role in establishing Colorado's first sanatorium for indigent consumptives.

Indeed, an American Jewish medical tradition of "caring for their own" extended back as far as 1654, when the first Jewish community in North America was formed when twenty-three Jews from Brazil first landed in New Amsterdam (New York). Even before the idea of the hospital had been conceived, some Denver Jews had sheltered impoverished Jews in their own homes. But the founding of NJH also reflected the desire of this early group of acculturated and affluent German Jews in Denver to demonstrate their commitment to American ideals and their value as loyal, productive American citizens. As Naomi Cohen has observed in *Encounter with Emancipation*, German Jews throughout America during this era believed philanthropy and charity were twin expressions of the strong civic responsibility of the Jew in American society at large. As members of a rising middle class who hoped to enlarge and enhance their position in American society, German Jews felt they could not help but gain "by chalking up an impressive record in philanthropy."[63]

These sentiments were certainly evident in a speech given at the dedication ceremonies of National Jewish Hospital on December 10, 1899, by board president Samuel Grabfelder of Kentucky. "Jews and Gentiles alike have been faithful in the work of ameliorating the conditions of humanity," he declared. "Without arrogance, however, I may be allowed to say that nowhere else is there a sanatorium devoted exclusively to the treatment of pulmonary diseases for the purpose of administering *alone* to those who are unable by reason of poverty, to purchase treatment of relief."[64]

Moreover, most early patients at the institution were East European immigrants, and the local German Jewish community, as did their counterparts around the United States, greeted their co-religionists with ambivalence. Although they viewed the plight of the East European Jews with sympathy and a sense of obligation, they also regarded these new immigrants, with their "outmoded" customs and Old World ways, as a source of embarrassment and possibly a threat to their own acceptance in American society. Abraham Karp, in *Golden Door to America*, described these mixed feelings succinctly: "The German Jews," he observed, "saw their Russian brethren as indigent refugees burdened by their barbaric culture. . . . They did not tire of informing their American neighbors that these were 'Different Jews.' At the same time they gave freely of their time and substance to help the Russian Jews become established, illuminated and Americanized."[65] Dr. Boris Bogen, who was one of those Russian immigrants and later became a leading Jewish American social worker, offered a firsthand memory of the era: "The rich, older Jews were quite upset by the strange mixture that was pouring in upon them from Eastern Europe and which by a generous giving of money they were trying to make American. There were Socialists of several varieties who, far from consenting to be made over, were resolved to help make America over."[66] In his own unique style, Charles Spivak clearly fit into the latter group.

From the beginning, many of the East European patients at NJH felt the administration treated them in a condescending manner and had little regard for many of their customs and religious observances. The absence of a kosher kitchen at NJH until 1923, for example, at the least reflected a lack of sensitivity to the traditions of many of those patients. An editorial in *The Denver Jewish Outlook* (the periodical published by Denver's early German Jewish community) in October 1904 argued that serving kosher meals to the patients at NJH would not be possible because tubercular patients needed a combination of meat, milk, and butter at all meals to restore their health.[67] This was, of course, a direct violation of Jewish dietary laws.

In addition to providing fine medical care, the NJH administration was also intent on acculturating and Americanizing the Jewish newcomers and provided English classes, vocational training, and civic instruction to that end. The goal, in part, was to transform the immigrants into upstanding American citizens with middle-class values of which the German Jews could be proud or, at the least, not ashamed. Many of the Jews of German descent who supported NJH had been born in America or were sufficiently integrated into U.S. society to view themselves as full Americans. As medical and immigration historian Alan Kraut has pointed out, "Medicine has been an important instrument employed by native-born Americans to assimilate immigrants into American society in a manner that would most effectively preserve the established order's cultural preferences and priorities."[68] This phenomenon was clearly played out on the NJH stage.

Influenced by Progressive-Era thought, which emphasized an efficient business model for running charitable institutions, while National Jewish Hospital gave its services free of charge, it also imposed firm rules governing patient admissions. NJH had introduced a revolutionary concept in tuberculosis treatment by offering free services to indigent consumptives, but its early admissions policies and types of treatment were largely in line with contemporary medical views. As a general rule, only patients with incipient tuberculosis were admitted to NJH. In addition to a formal application and medical examination by a physician appointed by the hospital, patients had to show proof of sufficient funds either to remain in Denver after discharge or to return to their original homes so they would not become a burden on the Denver community. In addition, patients could only remain at NJH for six months.[69]

The hospital's emphasis on limiting the length of stay and generally admitting only patients in the early stage of the disease reflected both the scarcity of hospital beds for consumptives at the time and the belief that attempting to treat advanced cases wasted time and money that could be more profitably directed toward patients who had a good chance of recovery. Certainly, many physicians such as Dr. Edward Trudeau felt sanatorium treatment was most successful with incipient cases.[70] At Philadelphia's White Haven sanatorium, Dr. Lawrence Flick advised against admitting "unsuitable" patients with advanced cases of tuberculosis because they had a depressing effect on other patients, disrupting morale and discipline.[71] Opened in 1895, just a few years before NJH, White Haven only accepted early-stage tuberculosis victims as patients, whom administrators felt could improve in six months and be considered rehabilitated.[72] Similarly, in the NJH's *First Annual Report* in 1900, President Grabfelder had stated that "[o]ur aim is to cure, not provide a last home for incurables."[73]

Charles Spivak's lifelong anti-elitist views were born in turbulent Tsarist Russia, nurtured in Philadelphia—the City of Brotherly Love—and brought to fruition in the wide-open atmosphere of the American West. Given Spivak's long-standing socialist and egalitarian convictions, his particular sympathy for the ill and the impoverished, and his strong connection to his fellow East European Jewish immigrants, his parting of the ways with the National Jewish Hospital administration becomes understandable. According to his good friend Dr. Boris Bogen, Spivak attempted to get the leaders of NJH to modify their rigid rules, which excluded so many needy persons. NJH refused and so launched Spivak on the course that would ultimately lead to the 1904 founding of the rival Denver Jewish Consumptives' Relief Society (JCRS), which treated patients in all stages of tuberculosis at no charge and catered to the religious traditions of its predominantly East European Jewish patients.[74]

The validity of this explanation is reinforced by Dr. Philip Hillkowitz, longtime president of the JCRS and Spivak's colleague and close friend: "The Sanatorium of the J.C.R.S. was established in 1904, at a time when all the current teaching and practice were in the direction of taking care of only the incipient cases of tuberculosis. In the pioneer days of the sanatorium movement, it was rank heresy to advocate the erection of sanatoria to treat both advanced and incipient cases. Dr. Spivak, actuated by his broad sympathy, which was an essential part of his character, spread his doctrines among the Jewish masses to help the advanced consumptive."[75]

Making treatment available for patients with advanced tuberculosis became a crusade for Charles Spivak through his leadership position at the JCRS. In May 1907 he presented a paper before the National Conference of Jewish Charities in Philadelphia, arguing that barring advanced cases from sanatorium treatment was not only inhumane but unscientific and medically unsound. Using biblical imagery, Spivak pointed out that advanced tuberculosis victims, who were patently "open cases" and the "fountain-head of all contagion" through their sputum and the microscopic droplets they spread through coughing and sneezing, were actually the ones in most need of isolation, as incipient cases were rarely a threat to public health. Refusal to admit consumptives in the advanced stage was a dire mistake: "Such a method," claimed Spivak, "is scientifically absurd, practically futile and morally brutal."[76]

Many years later, in 1925, Spivak offered a retrospective commentary in *The Denver Jewish News* on the early situation for tuberculosis sufferers who arrived in Colorado:

> The public commenced to show a rapidly developing pthisiophobia. Private boarding houses shut their doors against consumptives, all the hospitals came to an agreement not to admit tubercular patients to their wards. . . . Especially tragic was the fate of the Jewish consumptive at that time. Attracted to Denver in proportionately enormous numbers by the lure of the "Jewish Hospital" in which they expected to find a haven and a refuge among their own brothers, they arrived to find to their horror and dismay that the NJH admitted only incipient cases.[77]

Clearly, after more than a quarter century, the hospital's early policy still rankled.

Thus, Spivak's differences of opinion with NJH leaders reflected clashes in outlook over proper medical treatment as well as general antagonisms between the German and East European Jews in America. As Boris Bogen later perceptively remarked in a book on Jewish philanthropy, "At the turn of the century condescending attitudes and superiority feelings on the part of the givers of service aroused wide resentment and led to immigrant self-organization."[78] However, specific personal disagreements with particular individuals in Denver's German Jewish community no doubt also played a part in Spivak's distancing himself from NJH in its early years. Dr. Spivak had been a member of the International Order of B'nai B'rith in Philadelphia. When Spivak applied for membership in the Denver chapter in April 1905, he was rejected.[79] In Denver the lodge was founded in 1872 and for many years was composed largely of German Reform Jewish members. While some have seen Spivak's membership veto by the lodge as a rejection by the local German Jewish community,[80] it more likely reflected a personal quarrel with Alfred Muller, who was chair of the Board of Managers of National Jewish Hospital at the time and remained so until his death in 1911. After all, Spivak's relationship with the JCRS began in 1903, well before the B'nai B'rith incident. As a liberal, well-educated, highly cultured Jew, Spivak would probably have been well accepted in the group that made up Denver's B'nai B'rith.

The answer as to why Spivak was initially rejected by the B'nai B'rith and a possible explanation of some of the early antagonisms between the JCRS and NJH are possibly found in the "Atwood Colony Incident," retold later by New York social worker Chester Teller in his *Report on the Problem of Combined Poverty and Tuberculosis among the Jews in Denver, Colorado*, written in 1916. According to Teller, when Dr. Spivak moved to Denver from Philadelphia in 1896, a group of Jews from the latter city were emigrating to the tiny outpost of Atwood, Colorado, to join a Jewish agricultural colony there. Spivak, who as we have seen was a key figure in the national Jewish agricultural movement, understandably took a keen interest in the project. After settling in Denver, Spivak received complaints about the management of the Atwood colony from some former Philadelphia acquaintances. Spivak forwarded the complaints to the Denver B'nai B'rith, which had given financial and moral support to the new colony. Asked by the B'nai B'rith to report firsthand on the complaints, Spivak visited the colony with two other member of the fact-finding committee.[81]

Spivak signed the minority report, which concluded that the Atwood colony had been improperly managed. Alfred Muller, who became the executive secretary and chair of the provisional board of National Jewish Hospital in 1898, was then legal adviser to the Atwood colony and one of its prime promoters. As Teller pointed out, "For a number of years, likewise his name [Spivak's] was proposed to membership in the Denver Lodge of the I.O.B.B., but he was not elected to membership in this lodge until the year 1911, just subsequent to the death of Mr. Alfred Muller."[82] Seen in this light, it is likely that Spivak viewed his rejection by B'nai B'rith as a reflection of Muller's personal animosity rather than a rejection by the entire Jewish community. It is also probable that the tension between the two men exacerbated the discord between NJH and the JCRS in the early years. Until Muller's death, B'nai B'rith contributions went exclusively to NJH, as the lodge refused to donate any funds to support the JCRS. The B'nai B'rith minutes indicate that Muller was behind this early rejection of the JCRS.[83]

While the Jewish and general communities appreciated the work NJH carried out on behalf of poor tuberculosis patients, discontent over a number of the hospital's policies prompted a small group of Denver East European Jewish immigrants—many afflicted with tuberculosis—to make plans for the formation of another Jewish sanatorium. That sanatorium evolved into the Jewish Consumptives' Relief Society. The founders intended this new sanatorium to be more responsive to the needs of more traditionally oriented religious Jews as well as those with more advanced cases of tuberculosis. The details of the plans for the proposed institution are discussed in Chapter 5, but Dr. Charles Spivak became involved early on. In 1903, just a few years after NJH opened, a mass meeting was held in Denver's west side Jewish immigrant quarter to publicize the project. Three prominent Denver East European Jewish physicians—Dr. Philip Hillkowitz, Dr. Charles Spivak, and Dr. Adolph Zederbaum—were invited to address the well-attended fateful gathering, and their names would be intertwined with the JCRS for the rest of their lives. In fact, the three became fast friends, and Spivak's daughter Deena recalled that when she was young, "I don't think we ever had supper without one of them [Hillkowitz and Zederbaum"].[84] Dr. Hillkowitz described Spivak's initiation into the group of JCRS supporters: "Dr. Spivak, always in close touch with the unfortunate and the submerged, and deeply receptive of all things Jewish, was naturally called on as one of the speakers for that first public meeting. At the conclusion of the historic event, Dr. Spivak found himself secretary of a movement to solve the problems of the tuberculosis poor."[85]

5

The Genesis of the JCRS: Creating a New Type of TB Institution

> In a dingy room on West Colfax, on the 31st day of October, 1903, a small group of people, most of whom had at one time harbored the tubercle bacilli in their lungs, met for the purpose of devising means of how to help destitute consumptives in Denver. . . . A collection was made, and the magnificent sum of $1.10 was realized. . . . At a mass meeting held January 2, 1904, the society was permanently organized under the name of "The Jewish Consumptives' Relief Society," whose aim and object was defined to be "the relief of destitute consumptives in all stages of the disease."

This is how Dr. Charles David Spivak began his chronicle of the modest origins of the Jewish Consumptives' Relief Society (JCRS) in his secretary's report, published in the JCRS's *First Annual Report of 1905*.[1]

Spivak's close friend and colleague, JCRS president Dr. Philip Hillkowitz, described the progress of this small group of Jewish "poor dwellers of the Ghetto," as it enlarged its base to include prominent local doctors such as himself, the Russian-born Dr. Adolph Zederbaum, and Charles Spivak. Both Spivak and Hillkowitz were drawn to the new JCRS institution through a shared commitment to democratic socialist principles, as evidenced in Hillkowitz's remarks. "We are proud of the humble and lowly origins of our Society," he continued. "We rejoice in the fact that our beginning was distinctly a movement from below, not initiated by men of high economic or social standing."[2]

By the time the JCRS opened, Wilhelm Roentgen's discovery of the X-ray had helped revolutionize the treatment of tuberculosis by providing a valuable diagnostic tool. Within a few years, in 1907, another German, Clemens von Pirquet, added a skin test to the diagnostic arsenal in the war against the White Plague, so named for the white cheese-like material found in the lung cavities of tuberculosis victims. As the JCRS sanatorium developed, its leaders would share some optimistic contemporary convictions: that the spread of the disease was preventable by educating patients and isolating the afflicted from the general community and that tuberculosis was curable in many cases if caught early and if patients could be treated in a "proper" environment. Dr. Lawrence Flick of Philadelphia, one of the acknowledged leaders in the early American tuberculosis movement, declared, "If every consumptive in the land could at once be placed in a hospital, tuberculosis would be stamped out in a few years."[3] As Dr. Spivak later explained, "In the Sanatorium he [the patient] learns the best methods of regaining his health, and masters the rules of the game. Long after he is graduated he continues to apply the lessons he has learned in his alma mater, for the consumptive even after he is 'arrested' must look out for relapses and govern himself accordingly."[4]

On June 25, 1904, the JCRS was officially incorporated, with Rabbi Elias Hillkowitz, Mrs. Charles (Jennie) Spivak, and Mr. A. (Abraham) Kobey serving as signatories. Rabbi Hillkowitz was known as Denver's "dean" of Orthodox rabbis; Jennie, the only woman to serve as an incorporator, was the wife of Charles Spivak and was well-known in Denver as an educator, writer, and activist; and Abraham Kobey was an East European Jewish immigrant who served as a *sofer*, or scribe, in Denver's West Colfax Jewish community. His wife, Miriam, was a popular midwife, and his daughter, Rachel, was married to a Polish immigrant, Isaac Shwayder. In the early 1900s Isaac and his five sons founded a trunk company in Denver that

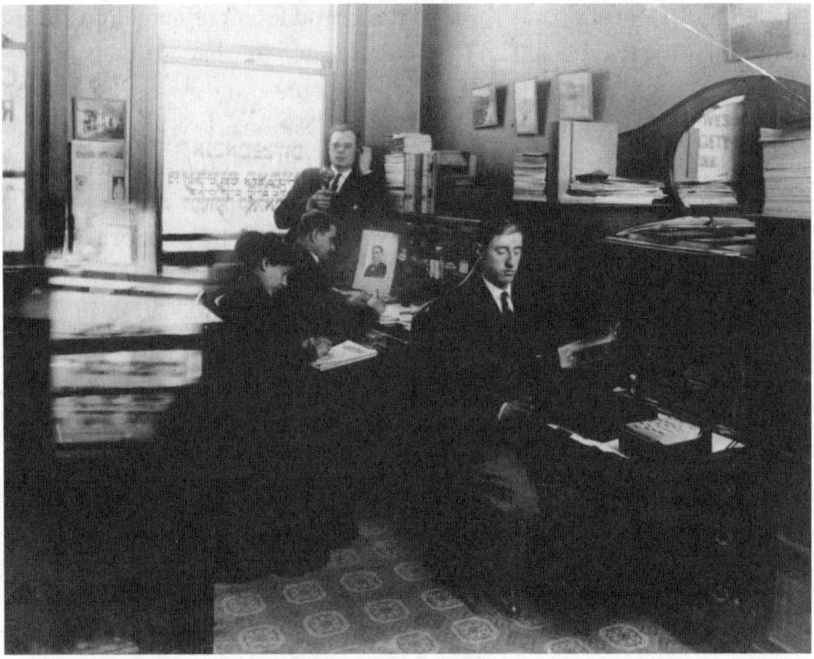

Dr. Charles David Spivak seated at the rear desk in the JCRS office, ca. 1910. Courtesy, Beck Archives, Special Collections, Penrose Library, University of Denver.

later became the internationally famous Samsonite Luggage Corporation. Less than a year after the idea for the alternative Jewish tuberculosis sanatorium was conceived, the JCRS was formally dedicated on September 4, 1904, a bright and sunny day that reflected the participants' optimism. Four days later the JCRS opened its doors to its first patients, six men and one woman, who were housed in inexpensive white, wooden tent-cottages to maximize their exposure to fresh air.[5]

When the JCRS admitted its first patients in 1904, Robert Speer was serving as Denver's mayor. Speer was a tuberculosis victim from Pennsylvania who had migrated to Denver's higher, dryer climate to "chase the cure." Most notably associated with the City Beautiful movement and the creation of many of Denver's beautiful parks and tree-lined boulevards, Speer aspired to turn the former mining camp into what he termed the "Paris of America." Another tuberculosis victim, Saco R. DeBoer, a prominent landscape architect from Holland, also contributed to the beautification of Denver's parks through the introduction of numerous flower beds and attractive trees. The JCRS was located in what was then considered the "country," in adjacent Jefferson County, and it was situated on twenty acres of land purchased for $5,000.[6] National Jewish Hospital was located approximately ten miles east of the JCRS on the opposite end of Colfax Avenue. That was probably simply a coincidence, but the symbolic irony of the opposing locations surely was not lost on the supporters of the two institutions.

The early JCRS campus featured a modest combination of seven tent-cottages and a central frame building, the latter a makeshift, even primitive edifice. It variously, if not always adequately, served as a kitchen, dining room, pantry, and linen closet and on cold evenings doubled as a library, den, and general recreation room. While the first central building was not an example of architectural beauty, as Dr. Spivak remarked, for a total cost of $317 one could hardly expect much splendor.[7] During the first three years, thirty-four canvas-type tents were donated by various organizations or individuals at a cost of $75 each. However, as the years passed, the negative effects of extremes of heat and cold on patients propelled the JCRS administration to erect several new buildings with modern indoor wards to supplement the tents. While the tents were extremely popular at first because of the medical emphasis on fresh air, by 1917 Dr. Spivak was declaring that "instead of a help to the patients, they [the tents] are a menace to them."[8]

Perhaps inspired by Mayor Speer's vision, the JCRS developed beautifully landscaped and well-maintained grounds, filled with a variety of trees and flowers, as well as a farm to provide milk, fresh eggs, poultry, and vegetables for the patients.[9] JCRS patients could stroll outdoors as part of their recovery plan; when looking to the west they often had a clear view of the famed snow-capped Rocky Mountains, which had earned Colorado the unofficial nickname "Switzerland of America." DeBoer, who served as Denver's official landscape architect from 1910 to 1931, later contributed to the JCRS plan, which included a central flower bed that ran the length of the main "avenue" between the sanatorium buildings. The JCRS minutes for February 9, 1921, indicate that the trustees authorized the payment of 50 percent of the "amount contracted on beautifying the ground."[10]

Unless a visitor had his or her own horse and carriage or an automobile, it was necessary to take the streetcar to the end of the line at

Colfax Avenue and Sheridan Boulevard (effectively the west boundary of Denver's west side immigrant neighborhood) and either walk the mile and a half distance to the JCRS or be picked up by a driver with a horse and wagon. For many years Spivak used a horse and buggy on his frequent visits to the JCRS before acquiring his own "machine," an old automobile that frequently required repairs.

The JCRS evolved into one of the most impressive of the Jewish immigrant self-help organizations and soon commanded a national reputation. Dr. Charles Spivak and Dr. Philip Hillkowitz worked in tandem at its helm for nearly a quarter century. Theirs was an interesting partnership. Hillkowitz was born in Russia but had immigrated to America with his parents as a young boy and had been educated in Cincinnati, where he graduated from Ohio Medical College in 1897. That same year he opened his practice in Denver, where he joined his parents and siblings who had moved to the Queen City earlier because of Rabbi Hillkowitz's asthma condition. In addition to his voluntary duties as president of the JCRS from 1904 until his death in 1948, Hillkowitz served as a professor of pathology at the Denver and Gross Medical College and held the positions of both state and City of Denver chemist. An early ardent Zionist, Hillkowitz helped found Denver's first Zionist organization and, as a well-known intellectual, was often seen riding a bicycle with a book propped up on the handlebars. He also served as vice president of Denver's Dante Society at the turn of the twentieth century. During World War I he served as a captain in the army medical corps. The brilliant doctor was said to have been fluent in fourteen languages.[11]

The two men obviously had much in common in their immigrant backgrounds, their interest in medicine and especially the treatment of tuberculosis, and their commitment to their fellow immigrants, but it was their different types of personalities that made them an effective team as advocates for the JCRS. One patient who knew both men in the early 1920s recalled that next to the magnetic personality of Dr. Spivak, Hillkowitz appeared soft-spoken, reserved, and almost naive to the realities of the world.[12] Spivak was witty, yet compassionate; fiercely intelligent, yet warm and highly accessible. In other words, the two physicians complemented each other. While many of the medical policies at the JCRS sanatorium reflected wider norms of tuberculosis treatment around the country, a number of significant innovations were introduced—many influenced by

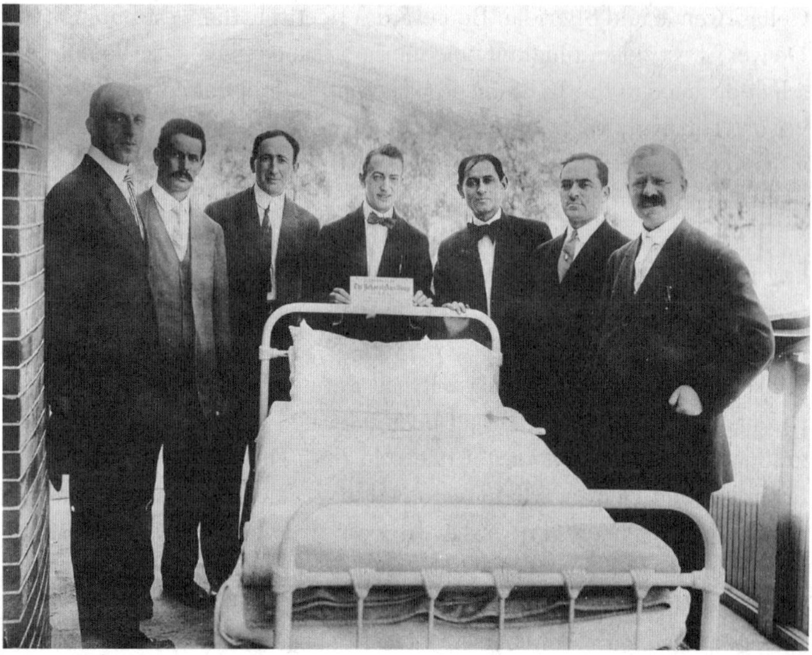

Many of the JCRS beds were sponsored by charitable contributions. This bed was dedicated in honor of the Yiddish poet Yehoash (Solomon Bloomgarden) in 1911. Left to right: Dr. Herman Schwatt, medical director; Abraham Judelovitz, a Denver builder and JCRS volunteer; Dr. Philip Hillkowitz, longtime president of the JCRS; Ben Frumess, Solomon Bloomgarden, Mr. Kulp, Dr. Charles David Spivak. Courtesy, Beck Archives, Special Collections, Penrose Library, University of Denver.

Spivak's particular outlook and his unusual sensitivity to the disease's psychological and emotional aspects.

Ethnic institutions like the JCRS helped ease immigrants' often difficult adjustment to a new life. Although the founding and development of the JCRS was a collective enterprise, Spivak wielded disproportionate influence by virtue of his energetic personality and broad knowledge. Under Spivak's influence the JCRS exhibited a rather unique blend of Old World traditions and modern progressive American norms and medical treatment. He served as a bridge between the past and future while honoring both. Spivak understood that emphasis on Jewish traditional celebrations would make the East European patients more comfortable and that happier patients made for healthier patients. "If he [the patient] feels at home in the place his recovery is hastened; otherwise it is retarded or prevented," he wrote.[13] In May 1906 Spivak approvingly recorded that "[t]he [recent] Passover Feast was celebrated this year with great eclat and enthusiasm. . . . The Seder was conducted in good old Orthodox fashion."[14]

As historian Hasia Diner observed in *Hungering for America,* ethnic food customs are connected closely with images of childhood and family and serve "as a mnemonic, an agent of memory."[15] Spivak's old friend from Philadelphia, the Russian immigrant Yiddish writer Leon Kobrin, prominently featured Jewish food culture in his 1927 novel about life in a fictional Lithuanian village.[16] For many immigrants groups, especially Jews, food and ethnic customs were intertwined. A significant number of Jewish patients at the JCRS viewed kosher food as central to their sacred observance. Although not all sanatorium patients were observant Jews, celebrating Jewish holidays and being served kosher meals were ways to preserve at least some forms of tradition. In his *Sixth Annual Report* in 1909, Spivak pointed proudly to the wholesome good food at the JCRS, which included traditional Jewish dishes such as Gefillte (stuffed) fish, Jauch mit Lokshen (soup with noodles), Tzimmes (a sweet carrot dish), and Gehakte Leber (chopped liver) and noted that "[s]uch a dietary is next in efficacy to the fresh air."[17] The JCRS, then, provided a nurturing environment while assisting the largely Jewish immigrant patient population to acculturate to mainstream American ideals.

Despite a disciplined daily treatment regimen, which assigned specific times for rest, light exercise, meals, and recreation, both Spivak and Hillkowitz emphasized a democratic style of operation at the JCRS. They proudly noted its support for and by the "masses," but some historians have viewed the sanatorium movement as a conscious effort to impose a middle-class social order on the working classes. Historian Georgina Feldberg, for example, has maintained that "between 1900 and 1925, TB offered a powerful rationale for the prescriptions that gave the middle class its shape and substance." Physicians supervising tuberculosis patients used the treatment of the disease as a tool of social reform that, according to Feldberg, "fused the goals of medical and social improvement."[18] As germ theory developed, the emphasis on sanitation and hygiene was seen as a valuable tool in preventing the disease, and public education was viewed as essential.[19] Major strides in bacteriology produced an era of scientific optimism, in which prevention offered the promise of eliminating disease.

However, as historian Nancy Tomes pointed out in her book *The Gospel of Germs*, in addition to elements of social control, concern about economic and social justice also emerged among middle- and upper-class Progressive-Era reformers who felt an obligation for the health of others.[20] Both elements were visible in Charles Spivak's work at the JCRS, but his sharply honed sense of responsibility for the ill and impoverished was primary. Undoubtedly, whether conscious or not, the JCRS under Spivak's aegis assisted in Americanizing the immigrant patients and imparted many middle-class values such as discipline, organization, and acceptable social practices. It discouraged patients from the unhealthy and "filthy" habit of spitting, a central tenet in the anti-tuberculosis crusade and what Tomes has termed "the worst of the mortal sins" in the "tuberculosis religion."[21] While spitting could spread germs, it was also considered uncouth by the upper classes. So, discouraging the habit had a dual motivation. A short article, for example, published in the JCRS *Sanatorium* in September 1907, highlighted best practices in the tuberculosis campaign and noted that the New York Board of Health had mounted a stereopticon exhibit in local parks in that city warning against the spread of tuberculosis through "bad hygiene, careless expectoration and crowded living."[22] As Feldberg has asserted, many physicians of a reform bent found in tuberculosis an opportunity for both fighting disease and inculcating middle-class values.[23]

In fact, prescriptive educational columns appeared regularly in the JCRS *Sanatorium* that were replete with educational advice for fighting the White Plague. A 1909 article authored by several leading American public health officials used imagery popular at the time and likened the tuberculosis germ to a seed planted by a farmer in "suitable soil." To prevent the body from becoming fertile "soil" for tuberculosis, people were encouraged to live and work in well-ventilated areas, eat nourishing food, and get adequate rest and fresh air. A central goal of the American tuberculosis crusade was to convince the public that tuberculosis was communicable and to discourage habits that spread the disease. Subtle instructions introduced middle-class values that emphasized cleanliness and orderliness and criticized "viscous personal habits" such as "intemperance" and use of tobacco.[24]

As a "modern" physician with a great respect for science, Spivak lobbied for many of the same goals in fighting tuberculosis. In the 1920s, for example, he penned a popular article written in a humorously affectionate style in the Jewish newspaper *The Forward* titled "Don't Crawl into a Clean Bed with Dirty Feet," aimed at promoting habits of cleanliness among East European immigrant workers.[25] Yet Spivak's socialist roots and affinity for the working classes were clearly evident. They enabled him to proudly validate the dignity of the institution's poor immigrant founders:

> The men who conceived the idea of organizing a national movement [the JCRS] for combating tuberculosis in all stages of its disease among those of our brethren who come to Colorado as to their haven of hope, differed in many respects from all organizers of any other existing national Jewish philanthropic institutions in the United States. There were no business men among them, no millionaires, lawyers or doctors—the usual figures in charitable enterprises. . . . They were simply workingmen and therefore had no rating in Bradstreet's, no show in Dunn's . . . nor the polish of the college-bred about them.[26]

Unlike many early Russian Jewish radicals who embraced universal world humanity but rejected "bourgeois" traditions, such as middle-class values and Jewish identity and religious observance, as the years passed Spivak increasingly gravitated to these ideals as well as toward middle-class respectability. In his work at the JCRS, Spivak's radical proclivities were channeled into what prominent social worker Dr. Boris Bogen termed "a new departure in Jewish Social Service in the United States."[27] Indeed, Spivak would have increasing influence on East European Jews in the American Jewish political and social scene as he moved from immigrant "outsider" to a position of local and national prominence.

The change in Jewish social service that Bogen referred to evolved from the initial clash between supporters of the National Jewish Hospital for Consumptives (NJH) and the JCRS. The NJH leaders warned initially that founding a second Jewish sanatorium in Denver would cause indigent consumptives to descend on Denver with charitable demands that would overwhelm the small Jewish community. They publicly voiced the opinion that the JCRS would be incapable of providing "proper" medical care for tuberculosis patients. In April 1904 Rabbi William Friedman of Denver's

German Jewish Reform Congregation Emanuel and a founder of NJH criticized the JCRS in an editorial in *The Jewish Outlook*. "The appeal of the JCRS," he maintained "extends an open invitation to the Jewish communities of the United States to send their penniless consumptives to Colorado. . . . The society cannot possibly benefit the incurable consumptives and is a dangerous menace to Colorado."[28] Friedman's remarks cut to the core of the debate about treating advanced cases of tuberculosis, questions concerning scientific charity and power issues within the American Jewish community. Yet Spivak took on Rabbi Friedman and the establishment to champion what he considered a good cause.

Spivak successfully argued his case before the National Conference of Jewish Charities. In establishing the JCRS, Spivak and the sanatorium's other leaders and supporters were in effect challenging the hegemony of the American German Jewish elite. Bogen perceptively described the situation: "Up to that time [the founding of the JCRS] it was taken for granted that the newcomers, or speaking more specifically, the Jews from Russia, were not only unable to contribute to the support of various [charitable] institutions, but were incapable of managing and directing their own agencies. Dr. Spivak more than anyone else, demonstrated the fallacy of that prejudice."[29] In other words, Spivak played a key role in transforming Jewish leadership from the German Jewish cohort to the East European newcomers. He utilized his personal charisma on behalf of the JCRS cause, turning the sanatorium into a world-renowned health institution as well as a symbolic cultural battleground for control of the American Jewish community.

Moreover, the JCRS paradigm would serve as an example for similar segments of the population in other American cities. Although the NJH and the JCRS remained in competition for years, the latter's reputation grew, as did the need for its services and its ability to sustain itself financially. By 1906 Dr. Hillkowitz was claiming that Rabbi Friedman's warnings had proven to be totally unfounded. "All those portentous predictions," he said, "of dire calamities—of flooding Colorado with consumptives, of lowering the price of real estate, of increasing racial prejudice, of quarantine against tuberculars—all these have long vanished as mist before Colorado sunshine."[30] Spivak's reputation within the established German Jewish community continued to rise as his medical and humanitarian work garnered increasing respect around the country.

Spivak continued to keep the issue of scientific charity before the public. During the Progressive Era, which roughly spanned the years 1900 to 1920, an atmosphere of reform pervaded developing American social policy. Although some historians have maintained that progressivism was too diffuse and amorphous to be properly considered a movement, others have maintained that during the Progressive Era a wide-reaching "progressive ethos," characterized by optimism and a firm belief in the efficacy of positive change primarily through education and "social engineering," affected large numbers of Americans.[31] These principles were often applied to public health initiatives, including tuberculosis treatment. Educating Americans about measures to prevent tuberculosis and "controlling" the behavior of victims became central aspects of the tuberculosis crusade.

Although he admired the educational and reform elements of contemporary Progressive-Era currents, Spivak, the trained physician and man of science, was critical of the wholesale application of business and scientific principles to charity. In an editorial written in 1907 he tried to reconcile the two, declaring that "[t]he present age is justly proud of its glorious records of brilliant discoveries and ingenious inventions so useful to mankind. Our progress in all lines of human endeavor has been made possible by the application of scientific methods." At the same time, he declared that "we are naturally repelled by that type of professional charity official who styles himself scientific" and concluded regretfully that "the personal and human element is entirely lacking" and that instead, charity should "be dispensed in the spirit of the good, old charity or as a writer aptly said, let it be 'charity of the heart, not of the head.'" Spivak clearly rejected the popular contemporary emphasis on scientific charity. To that end, he maintained that JCRS patients should be made to feel at home as part of a "sanatorium family."[32]

Often characterized as the "guiding genius" behind the JCRS, Dr. Spivak placed his personal imprint and outlook on virtually every aspect of the JCRS, which according to Spivak rested on a "humanitarian" policy as its underlying raison d'être. The "individualization of cases is our guiding principle," he wrote, "in treating patients from the incipient stage to the advanced emergency cases."[33] As JCRS secretary, Spivak signed an individual welcoming letter to each new patient, inviting the patient to make him- or herself at home. He confidently informed them that "[e]verything will be prepared to receive you and make you comfortable."[34] His daughter

Deena Spivak Strauss recalled that a bouquet of flowers and a basket of fruit were placed in each new patient's room.[35] In addition, Spivak took careful minutes of the JCRS board meetings, beginning in 1903 when the sanatorium was in its initial planning stages until his death in 1927. The minutes begin first in his elegant copperplate handwriting and then, as time passed, appear as a typescript with his distinctive signature appearing at the end.[36]

Spivak noted that the JCRS administration "encouraged the patients to come to them with their troubles, little or big, and speak without reservation or hesitation."[37] This policy helped him earn the sobriquet "Papa Spivak." The role of secretary at the JCRS was what today we would term executive director. Spivak supervised general and business operations, as well as fundraising, and contributed regularly to the institution's publications. In his fundraising appeals he was forceful, and he did not hesitate to manipulate heartstrings.

In an early solicitation, for example, he informed potential contributors that "[i]t is your duty to join our organization as a member or contributor. The charitable work that you are invited to support morally and materially, according to your influence and means, is the only one of its kind. It cannot fail to appeal to everybody whose heart is not calloused and whose imagination is vivid enough to reproduce before his eyes the tragedies of the struggling and suffering of hundreds and thousands of Jewish consumptives."[38] Spivak's colleague Dr. Philip Hillkowitz recalled his friend's public relations efforts on behalf of the JCRS and maintained that "[a]s a publicist he [Spivak] had no equal."[39] His persuasive style is clearly evident, and as a public health educator and fundraiser, Spivak was making good use of business and public relations techniques in the new field of advertising.[40]

Spivak's "propaganda," as it was called at the JCRS, or fundraising solicitations as we would label it today, resulted in wide support for the JCRS from contributors throughout the United States, particularly members of the working class. In the first year of the sanatorium's existence, a little over $7,000 was raised. In 1906 nearly $32,000 was collected, and the numbers continued to grow yearly.[41] Small contributions, sometimes as little as twenty-five cents, were recorded over and over again, undoubtedly influenced by Spivak's socialist leanings and his emphasis on relying on the "masses" for support.[42]

Dr. Spivak personally supervised most early fundraising activities at the sanatorium, overseeing the work of a number of "field secretaries" who canvassed the nation in search of financial support for the JCRS. Spivak's wife, Jennie, while not an official worker, was helpful in fundraising. A short time after the JCRS opened, Jennie made a presentation to the Chicago chapter of the National Council of Jewish Women, which led the organization's national president, Hannah Solomon, to push the well-known women's group to support the sanatorium.[43]

One of Spivak's most successful workers was Anna Hillkowitz, sister of Dr. Philip Hillkowitz and a Denver librarian. She took a leave of absence from her public library position in 1906 to collect money for the JCRS. Within just six months she visited nearly forty cities, and her fascinating correspondence with Dr. Spivak survives. Anna Hillkowitz often turned to Dr. Spivak for advice and moral support. When Hillkowitz wrote Spivak in May 1906 concerning her hope to approach a number of wealthy Jews for contributions, Spivak firmly replied, "I think you should entirely abandon the idea of making any strenuous efforts to meet our rich brethren. If our Institution is to be a people's institution, it should be supported by the people only. Let us collect our moneys in dollars and quarters."[44] In the letter, Spivak summed up the essence of his philosophy that still bore the imprint of his socialistic roots: the East European Jewish immigrant masses were capable of supporting and running their own "democratic" institutions without the aid of wealthy, often condescending Jewish capitalists. In his mind, leadership skills were clearly and emphatically not only found among the acculturated German Jews. The emphasis on numerous small donations proved an economically successful policy for several decades, but after Spivak's death and changes brought about by the Great Depression, larger donations by wealthy individuals helped keep the institution afloat.

Spivak often complimented Hillkowitz on her success. After she had received a check for $100 in Oklahoma, where he noted she had "brought in the dough," he enthused "[h]urray! Three cheers for the Field Secretary of the JCRS. You have done wonderfully well."[45] When she complained about the challenges of raising funds on a visit to Rochester, New York, Spivak observed with his usual humor and optimism: "I am by this time accustomed to hearing your complaints about the inhabitants of the various cities in the East, and yet after you are through with a city you nevertheless succeed in turning out their pockets, so I do not feel blue about your blue letters."[46] In other letters Spivak wished her a "Kosher *Pesach*" (Passover) and an "easy fast" before the solemn Jewish holiday Yom Kippur.[47]

Anna Hillkowitz was joined in early JCRS fundraising efforts by Russian Jewish immigrant Jacob Marinoff, later a noted Yiddish humorist and editor of the popular Yiddish humor weekly *The Big Stick*. Based in New York City, a key source of fundraising for the JCRS, under Spivak's supervision Marinoff concentrated on approaching Jewish fraternal orders, working-class organizations, and the numerous JCRS ladies' auxiliaries in countless cities around the country such as Chicago, St. Louis, New York, and Baltimore. Marinoff often placed JCRS charity boxes at New York City workshops, and in the first fifty-three of these boxes, a collection of $18.25 was proudly noted.[48] He did somewhat better among union organizations, and a January 1907 article in *The Sanatorium* noted that he had collected $25 from the United Garment Workers of America, $5 from the Children's Jacket Maker's Union, $8 from the Russia Poland Young Men's Association, and $75 from the Paper Cigarette Maker's Union.[49] While these sources of income were modest, Spivak looked upon them with approval as further demonstration of the generosity and support of the primarily Jewish workers.

In addition to supervising fundraising and publicity, Spivak was also centrally involved in medical treatment at the JCRS. While Spivak treated JCRS patients with gastrointestinal problems, a medical superintendent was hired to supervise the daily medical program, although Spivak had a voice in this area as well. For the first eight years Spivak served as executive director at no charge before he was persuaded to take a modest salary. In addition to his "secretarial" duties, Spivak volunteered his services as chair of the JCRS Admissions and Dismissions Committee and as a member of the Executive Committee, the Medical Advisory Board, and the Press and Propaganda Committee, which oversaw public relations.[50]

Sanatorium hospitals such as the JCRS and NJH became more common in America after 1900. As Georgina Feldberg has noted, "Sanatoria came to dominate the turn-of-the-century medical campaign against tuberculosis" and to build resistance against the disease through education and healthy living in an effort to regenerate the immune system through a program consisting of moderate exercise, good food, and fresh air.[51] In the absence of a vaccine to prevent the disease or a medication to cure it, emphasis was placed on making the individual "host" resistant to tuberculosis or preventing a relapse.

Early on, Spivak observed that "[o]ur [JCRS] patients are mainly recruited from those who, having been weakened by working in the congested districts of large cities, in factories and in workshops, have contracted the dread disease consumption."[52] A report written by a New York social worker emphasized that crowded urban tenement buildings were incubators for tuberculosis: "The Plague lives in darkness and filth—filth in halls, over walls and floors, in sinks and closets . . . rooms here have held death ready and waiting for years."[53] Dr. Hillkowitz echoed the popular contemporary emphasis on the need for sanatoriums to counteract undesirable urban conditions and maintained, "While we are anxiously waiting for the specific remedy to cure this disease, the best possible form of treatment, especially for the poor, is in a Sanatorium, where the patient is taught how to live the right kind of life, eat the proper food and be under gentle discipline and instruction so as to benefit his health and promote his recovery."[54]

Similarly, a 1908 article in *The Sanatorium* emphasized that "proper regulation" of the lives and treatment of tuberculosis victims could "only be carried out efficiently in special institutions. Hence we see the establishment of sanatoria for tuberculosis all over the United States." Acknowledging that a level of regimentation was necessary for recovery, the author, probably Dr. Spivak, emphasized that the JCRS carried out a policy of "science tempered by humanity." Moreover, "the word 'charity' is never mentioned."[55] Spivak's policy of "science tempered by humanity" reflected his ability to reconcile contradictions between scientific medical thought and his religious and social convictions. Spivak firmly believed that responsibility for caring for the ill extended to the most severe cases. Still, he acknowledged the limits of medical treatment for tuberculosis patients and the possibility of relapse even in arrested cases. He noted that "[a] certain number of patients who have undergone some repairs at our Sanatorium during the previous years came back . . . for further patching. We have never claimed, as other institutions do that we can make them 'as good as new.' "[56]

The JCRS sanatorium grew out of a long historical tradition of caring for consumptives. The first known example of an institution featuring open-air treatment of tuberculosis was the Royal Sea Bathing Infirmary, established in 1791 in Margate, England, by a Quaker physician. However, most American sanatoriums of the late nineteenth and early twentieth centuries were patterned after the German model of open-air treatment, where patients were located in a rural environment away from crowded cities. A tuberculosis open-air sanatorium founded in the late 1850s in the mountains of Silesia, Germany, by Dr. Hermann Brehmer emphasized constant fresh air and forced feeding for all tubercular patients. Brehmer's success in attracting patients inspired other physicians to follow his path. Sunlight or heliotherapy as an effective antidote for life in dank, congested urban neighborhoods also came to be a popular part of treatment at many American sanatoriums. This image of tenement living seemed to embody the tuberculosis threat for Progressive reformists. According to many tuberculosis specialists, sunlight destroyed bacteria and invigorated tuberculosis victims.[57] Several photographs of early JCRS patients feature men and women stripped to their underclothes stretched out on outdoor porches in lounge chairs or cots to maximize their exposure to sunlight's supposed health-giving properties.

Diet for tuberculosis patients was another prime example of the manner in which the JCRS adhered to the accepted emphasis on healthy food, which included large quantities of fresh milk, eggs, and meat but also incorporated respect for Jewish dietary laws. In his first secretary's report, Spivak noted that "milk, eggs and meat are the main factors in dealing with the disease." Therefore, he reported, "[w]e buy the best in the market—best cuts of Kosher meat, which is always higher than *Trepha* [non-kosher]; we give our patients the freshest eggs, milk and butter obtainable."[58] Hillkowitz reinforced Spivak's words, noting that "[o]ur Sanatorium is likewise unique in its culinary department, which is conducted along Kosher lines. The food is prepared in the way the patients have been accustomed to, with all the local color, the trimmings and frills of their own home."[59]

Spivak, along with Hillkowitz and Zederbaum, felt that offering observant Jewish patients a kosher diet would predispose them to recovery because of the positive psychological aspect of allowing them to maintain their religious practices. The three physicians were ahead of their time in appreciating the psychological factor in combating illness. In an article published in the JCRS *Sanatorium* in 1908, Dr. Zederbaum reinforced this position. In a veiled reference to the food policy at NJH he argued,

"It is mere nonsense to claim that a sick person cannot thrive on Jewish meat and delicacies. . . . [A]t the Sanatorium of the JCRS dairy articles never appear together with meat."[60] As East European Jews themselves, the three doctors understood the feelings of inferiority and resentment some of the NJH's policies had engendered and the potential deleterious affects on tuberculosis patients who, according to Hillkowitz, exhibited "a particularly sensitive nature."[61]

Therefore, as proscribed by Jewish law, kosher meat and milk products were never mixed together at the JCRS. Eggs, considered an especially effective tool in the food arsenal in the battle against tuberculosis, appeared frequently on the daily menu at the JCRS but were recommended in modest amounts compared to those at many other institutions. A weight gain to counteract the "wasting" effects of the disease was considered desirable in Denver and across the country, and meat, milk, butter, and eggs built resistance in the view of experts. At the Nordrach Ranch sanatorium in Colorado Springs, which was strongly influenced by the German model, patients were subjected to "disciplined gluttony" by director Dr. John E. White and "were not allowed to leave the table until every morsel was eaten and every drop was consumed." One patient at the institution recalled having to consume twenty-eight raw eggs daily as part of her routine.[62] At Trudeau's sanatorium at Saranac Lake the regimen was more moderate, but the patients typically consumed at least five raw eggs a day, as was also common at both NJH and the JCRS.[63] Similarly, at Philadelphia's White Haven sanatorium, Dr. Flick approvingly reported that "[o]ne man had seventeen glasses of milk and eight raw eggs yesterday and another fourteen and eight."[64]

Even the entertainment provided at the JCRS was geared toward the cultural interests of East European immigrants, with a library, for example, well-stocked with Yiddish as well as English books and periodicals. Early on, a Yiddish section had been incorporated in *The Sanatorium*. Yiddish poems and plays were often published in the magazine, and a serialized drama by the well-known Yiddish playwright Leon Kobrin appeared in both Yiddish and English versions in a 1907 issue of *Sanatorium*. Kobrin was the politically radical immigrant who Dr. Spivak had treated for a hand injury in Philadelphia in the early 1890s. Perhaps because of his longtime friendship with Spivak, Kobrin was persuaded to compose a play titled *The Rescue* especially for the JCRS publication. An editorial in *The*

Sanatorium, probably penned by Spivak, described the play as a "brilliant portrayal of the life of the consumptive" that ably described "the psychology of the consumptive, the anxiety of the relatives, the grinding poverty of the factory worker."[65]

Spivak played a central role in the Yiddish culture that permeated the early JCRS, and he was perhaps best known internationally in the East European Jewish community for the Yiddish dictionary he coauthored with the well-known Yiddish author Solomon Bloomgarden, who went by the pen name Yehoash. The Yiddish dictionary was published in New York in 1911, "containing All the Hebrew and Chaldaic (Aramaic) Elements of the Yiddish Language Illustrated with Proverbs and Idiomatic Expressions." A prominent ad for the dictionary appeared in a 1911 issue of the JCRS *Sanatorium*, proclaiming that the volume was "Just Ready" and that it had been compiled by Dr. C. D. Spivak and Sol Bloomgarden (Yehoash). The price for the volume was $2.50.[66]

According to Deena Spivak Strauss, the dictionary was composed at the Spivak dining room table, where Spivak and Bloomgarden worked painstakingly on the manuscript as their wives, Jennie and Flora, hovered in the background. Whenever a local woman came in to clean the house, Spivak stood next to the table to make sure none of the notes for the dictionary that littered the table were moved.[67] Spivak noted that the publication of the 340-page Yiddish dictionary helped make him a household name within the Jewish community. When Spivak traveled to Poland in 1920 on a humanitarian mission on behalf of East European Jews, his reputation as the author of the popular dictionary preceded him, and he was treated as a dignitary by the local Polish Jewish community.[68]

The Lithuanian-born Bloomgarden had contracted tuberculosis on the East Coast and arrived in Denver in 1899 to "chase the cure." He eked out a living taking on odd clerking jobs, all the while composing poetry. Through his friendship with Dr. Charles Spivak, Bloomgarden became active in the early JCRS, using his writing talents to help publicize the work of the Jewish sanatorium. A 1908 article titled "The Yehoash Receptions," which appeared in the JCRS *Sanatorium*, reported that Yehoash's East Coast tour to raise funds for the JCRS was very successful. Praising Bloomgarden, the article stated: "At the sacrifice of personal interests and even of his health he was braving the rigors of the eastern climate to preach the message of the J.C.R.S. to help the unfortunate consumptives."[69]

The sensitive poet soon became a member of the JCRS Press and Propaganda Committee. Bloomgarden also worked with Spivak and another friend, Jacob Marinoff, on *The Sanatorium*, which included not only reports and statistics related to the JCRS but medical advice, human interest stories, and poetry and literature as well. Both Bloomgarden and Marinoff served as members of the JCRS Board of Directors from its beginning in 1904.[70]

In 1913 Marinoff wrote to Spivak about a "blow out" celebration honoring Yehoash in New York City. He informed Spivak that they would be rushing souvenir programs for the event by special delivery to Spivak and Yehoash's other friends in Denver. Marinoff also made reference to a big affair at Carnegie Hall for the "eventful gathering of Jewish people, to do honor to a *landsman* [fellow countryman]." "Tickets are practically *all sold,*" enthused Marinoff, "and at fancy prices at that."[71] Although this is unclear, it is possible that the event was a fundraiser for the JCRS.

Bloomgarden also worked on his Yiddish translation of the Bible during his residence and treatment in Denver. That work was not published until after his death in 1927, the same year Spivak died.

Environmental issues, particularly overall climate and fresh air, were considered another set of essential tools in fighting tuberculosis. They were utilized to help susceptible individuals resist invasion from the tubercle germ by increasing respiratory efficiency and, indirectly, improving nutrition by increasing patients' appetites. Trudeau had made open-air therapy so popular through his Saranac Lake sanatorium model that Hillkowitz could assert: "The benefits of open air life in tents are too well known to everybody; I need not, therefore point out here, the reasons for adopting this form of treatment for tuberculosis. Our patients have done remarkably well, although the majority were advanced cases."[72]

Although patients were soon housed in more comfortable indoor wards, several years later Spivak was still touting Colorado as "the best climate for consumptives and even they who are not cured are in many ways benefited in Denver."[73] It is obvious that many eastern physicians clearly agreed with Spivak. One Boston doctor, for example, sent a Jewish patient with "General Pulmonary Tuberculosis" to Denver in 1904 with a note stating, "I sincerely recommend him to Denver, Colorado as there is no cure for him in the Eastern States."[74] The "great outdoors" was emphasized for tuberculosis patients, and suburban sites with agricultural potential were common for both European and American sanatoriums. Spivak lauded the fields of alfalfa and shady trees on the JCRS grounds as well as the benefits of Colorado's fresh, clean air and high altitude. He particularly praised the view of the Rocky Mountains afforded to JCRS patients. "The vision is an inspiring one," he wrote," and must be of benign influence in raising the spirits of our patients—a psychical factor of great moment in the improvement of their health."[75]

Unsurprisingly, considering Spivak's long-standing ties with the Jewish agriculture movement, he strongly supported an evolving JCRS farm, which eventually provided patients with fresh eggs, milk, and fruits and vegetables. Professor Simon Simpkins, a graduate of the Baron de Hirsch Agricultural School and Cornell University, was hired in 1904 to direct the horticultural and agricultural activities at the JCRS.[76] The Baron de Hirsch Agricultural School had been established by de Hirsch, a Bavarian-born Jew who had been interested in involving Jews in farming and removing them from city ghettos. Spivak had been closely involved with the concept in his Alliance colony and Philadelphia days, where he first became acquainted with Simpkins. Spivak undoubtedly had a hand in hiring Simpkins, and the farm at the JCRS no doubt satisfied some of Spivak's own early longing to "work the land."

Spivak seems to have taken a special interest in the farm's progress and happily reported that by 1906 the JCRS hennery and the small cow herd not only supplied patients with nutritious food but also allowed some of the healthier residents to perform light manual work out of doors. "The day will soon come," he predicted, "when every egg consumed will come from our hennery, and not only will we have enough cows to supply all the milk needed by our steadily increasing institution, but all milk products, as cream, butter, cheese, buttermilk, etc., will be manufactured on the premises."[77]

In addition to the accepted three-prong approach to tuberculosis treatment that focused on diet, fresh air, and rest as the prescription for "chasing the cure," as the years passed, surgical intervention to treat tuberculosis patients was introduced. The JCRS was a pioneer in this area. The goal of the operation was to "rest" the affected lung(s) to allow it to recover. Artificial pneumothorax, for example, was a procedure that injected air into the cavity between the lungs and chest walls, collapsed the lung, and prevented patients from taking a full breath.[78] Introduced in America in 1898 at the annual meeting of the American Medical Association, the procedure did not become well-known in the United States until pneumothorax machines were perfected around 1910. It was generally reserved for patients who had not responded well to the more common and far less invasive therapy, for the procedure could be both dangerous and painful. Still, by the late 1920s it became popular because a number of physicians claimed marked improvement for their patients as a result of pneumothorax.[79] Once the procedure became accepted, about a quarter of the patients at tuberculosis sanatoriums were subjected to the "collapse" therapy, which was supplemented in the 1930s by thoracoplasty, a procedure in which several ribs were removed to limit lung mobility.[80] The JCRS secured its own pneumothorax machine in 1911, soon after the device was perfected. From then until the late 1940s thousands of procedures were performed, nearly 1,400 in 1948 alone.[81]

Spivak devoted considerable time to the JCRS, but he also managed to keep up a busy medical practice at his home-based office at 1421 Court Place, at the edge of downtown Denver. The doctor inspired confidence in both his private patients and those he visited at the JCRS; he was "a man who would see you through all the way."[82] However, the Spivaks lived modestly because Charles's private practice suffered from the many hours he spent each week at "The San." His devotion to the patients became legendary. According to Deena Spivak Strauss, during Denver's famous blizzard of 1913, he became very concerned that the JCRS patients would be short of food staples because the snow had prevented normal deliveries from getting through. Inspired by the winters he had spent in Russia as a young boy and with his typical creativity and determination, he hit upon a solution. Although in his early fifties, Spivak donned a pair of snowshoes and carried a large sack of flour from his downtown home for the nearly five-mile trip to the JCRS sanatorium grounds so the cook could bake bread. His daughter also recalled that once he arrived home without the new winter overcoat his family had insisted he purchase; he had given it to a patient he felt needed it more than he did.[83]

Deena Strauss also remembered that when she was young she would often accompany her father on his visits to JCRS patients on weekends. In one pocket he carried candy treats to keep Deena occupied, and in the other pocket Spivak carried a little notebook in which he jotted down shopping requests the patients made. When he went home and into "town," he would make the purchases and deliver them to the patients on his next trip to the sanatorium.[84]

In Denver, Spivak continued to exhibit a contradictory and evolving religious persona. In his first secretary's report he concluded his address before the audience at the JCRS annual meeting by saying: "[W]hen I stand thus, with a heart palpitating with joy and exultation, the religious fervor of my young days flares up in my breast, and involuntarily, the old and beautiful benediction comes to my lips, 'Blessed be He who hath kept us in life and hath preserved us, and hath enabled us to reach this season.'"[85] Spivak was certainly referring to his early days in the home of his Orthodox Jewish parents, where he was raised in a traditional Jewish household and was a yeshiva student. The "Shechechyanu" is a traditional Jewish prayer of gratitude to the Almighty that has been recited by Jews for millennia. While Spivak had discarded many of his early Jewish traditions in his aspiration to become first a culturally assimilated Russian and then a "hundred percent American," some of his early Jewish religious observances gradually returned, although he appears to have been selective in which ones he chose to follow. Deena Strauss made a telling observation when she commented, "Papa had a religion all his own."[86] His granddaughter later echoed her mother's thoughts when she asserted, "Papa was a deeply religious man, but [he] didn't do everything by the book."[87]

In an article titled "Dr. C. D. Spivak, the Synagogue Jew," written by Rabbi Charles Kauvar after Spivak's death, Kauvar, the longtime spiritual leader of Denver's traditional Beth HaMedrosh Hagodol (BMH) Synagogue, reviewed Spivak's increasing Jewish commitment and "spiritual growth." Through their common devotion to the JCRS cause, Spivak and Kauvar became close friends over the years. Kauvar stated, "For a quarter of a century, I was privileged to watch the return of this distinguished son of Israel to his people. When I first knew him, this many-sided, versatile man of science gave his best energies to world movements but did not heed the call of the Synagogue."[88]

The newfound freedom Spivak encountered in America may have been the key to his increased religiosity. In Russia, opposition to religion had been intertwined with opposition to authority. As Spivak's contemporary, printer Gregory Weinstein, later recalled in his memoirs, "The youth of Russia was aflame with the spirit of rebellion against the authority of Church and State. . . . We became estranged from the faiths of our fathers.

. . . [L]ike zealots of a new religion, we discarded everything—valuable as well as valueless of the old teaching."[89] In the United States, where all citizens were free to observe religion as they saw fit and religion was separated from the political state, many came to find observance more appealing on at least a cultural level.

Rabbi Kauvar was in a position to observe Spivak firsthand, and it appears that initially there was some disagreement between the two men on the desirable degree of Jewish observance at the JCRS. For many years Kauvar regularly attended JCRS board meetings, at which he used his influence to ensure that Jewish traditions were observed at the institution. In June 1909, for example, Kauvar reaffirmed his great respect for the sanatorium administration and noted that the kosher kitchen "stamps it 'Jewish.'" At the same time he complained that office work conducted on Saturday, the Jewish Sabbath, violated Jewish law. He urged that office workers increase their weekday hours to avoid the situation. The minutes record that Dr. Spivak "said the observance of the Sabbath appeals to him" but insisted he would oppose the introduction of additional new stringencies.[90]

In addition to his longtime love for Yiddish, Spivak began to regard Hebrew as the language of what was sacred in Judaism. He began devoting more time to studying Hebrew texts, which he often incorporated into his writings. He was also reconnecting personally with Jewish observances. According to one source, Spivak paid dues to every local synagogue in Denver, which numbered at least a dozen during his residence; he conducted a traditional Passover Seder for JCRS patients every year; and in his home he brought in a new set of separate Passover dishes each year so his family would be following the traditional Jewish *halacha,* or law.[91]

Rabbi Kauvar observed of Spivak that as time went by, "because of his spiritual contacts the idealism of his youth broke through the crust of materialism," and "he was beginning to judge all things with the Jewish perspective." Dr. Spivak joined the BMH Synagogue, which Kauvar credited in part for Spivak's reconnection with the traditional Jewish community, and he noted that Spivak occasionally delivered popular sermons at the BMH and other local venues. Kauvar recalled in particular one sermon delivered at the B'nai B'rith Lodge in support of a Jewish Theological Seminary fundraising campaign, in which Spivak spoke out against contemporary assimilationist tendencies—particularly among former Orthodox Jewish immigrants like himself who had abandoned their faith and practices in the rush for societal acceptance and financial success. Kauvar quoted Spivak, the self-proclaimed early agnostic and political radical, as later maintaining that "our [the Jewish people's] great claim to the gratitude of mankind is that we gave to the world the word of God, the Bible, our sole *raison d'etre.*"[92]

On another occasion Kauvar recounted that Spivak declared to a group of scientists and professionals that "the older I get, the more I am convinced that if a new scientific theory is promulgated which finds no suggestion in the Scriptures we ought to doubt the theory, not the Bible." Kauvar poignantly recalled that in his last conversation with Dr. Charles Spivak before he passed away, just a few weeks before Spivak made his final trip to New York for radiation treatment, he asked Kauvar in Yiddish: "*Rebbi, Ich forh up heint. Git mir eier brocho*" (My rabbi, I am leaving today. Give me your blessing).[93]

At the same time, Jennie Spivak seems to have been undergoing her own religious/social/political transformation. By the late 1890s, as a budding writer, she was contributing articles to the Philadelphia *Jewish Exponent.* Among their common interests, Jennie and Charles Spivak had always shared an attraction to Jewish farming endeavors. In an essay published in August 1899, Jennie recounted in glowing terms a recent Sabbath visit she had made to the Jewish agricultural colony of Alliance, New Jersey, whose members were predominantly traditional in their Jewish observance. In fact, one Jewish newspaper reported of Alliance, "Sabbath observance is so general that we could not get a farmer to begin hitching a horse until darkness set in."[94]

Jennie Charsky Spivak, the early political radical of whom Spivak's colleague Dr. Michael Ball had noted in Philadelphia in 1893 that "marriage and religion are all mockery in her eyes,"[95] was a seemingly contented wife a few years later who offered a very positive account of the Friday evening Jewish Sabbath observance at Alliance. She wrote approvingly of the time when Jewish families gathered "to greet the beautiful bride, the Sabbath, the day of rest"—complete with the traditional lighting of the candles by the women to usher in the Sabbath, white tablecloths and the traditional *challah* bread gracing the tables, and the men reciting the Friday evening prayer service. The early universalist also worried that other citizens might, "either from love or hatred, wish to obliterate [the Jewish] distinctiveness."[96]

As both Charles and Jennie Spivak matured, refined, and sometimes redefined their ideological outlooks as they entered their middle years, so did the JCRS. When the JCRS was described as exhibiting "a policy of science tempered with humanity,"[97] the description was appropriate for Charles Spivak himself, a man of intense contradictions who ultimately helped save thousands of lives and played a leading role in the battle to conquer tuberculosis. A man of many talents, Spivak—the early political revolutionary and proponent of Progressive Enlightenment thought—was moving into the social, medical, political, and even religious mainstream, all the while continuing to exhibit his own idiosyncratic style and outlook.

In a 1909 editorial in the JCRS *Sanatorium*, Spivak looked back with satisfaction on the institution's first five years. "The phenomenal rise and rapid growth of the Jewish Consumptives' Relief Society has been the marvel of all students of philanthropy," he asserted. "Starting with an initial fund of $1.10, it has within the short space of five years evolved into one of the foremost national organizations counting close to 20,000 members and contributors. Without depending on wealthy endowments or rich bequests, it has appealed directly to the masses of Jewish people native as well as immigrant, and by virtue of mere strength of numbers has become the most popular and widely known institution in American Jewry."[98] The same could be said of Charles Spivak, who had arrived in the United States a quarter century earlier as a penniless immigrant. By 1910 his reputation as a physician and at the JCRS had made him a well-known figure in medical, immigrant, and social service circles around the country.

6

Becoming a Westerner

The early discovery of gold in Colorado and the coming of the railroads were central to the transformation of Denver from a wilderness to a burgeoning metropolis, but the pivotal impact of tuberculosis on the area should not be underestimated. The search for health that focused on tuberculosis and other respiratory ailments was critical to the economic and population growth of the Mile High City in the first decades of the twentieth century, perhaps nowhere more visible than in the Jewish community. Although a handful of cities in the United States established specifically Jewish sanatoriums, Denver was the only city in the country to boast two national Jewish tuberculosis treatment centers. Following the opening of National Jewish Hospital (NJH) and the Jewish Consumptives' Relief Society (JCRS), the modest number of around 1,500 Jewish Coloradoans in 1897 ballooned to close to 15,000 by 1912.[1]

By the time the JCRS entered its second decade, the tuberculosis movement had gained significant momentum as a public health campaign, and Dr. Charles David Spivak was a fixture on the Denver and American landscape. In his tenth annual secretary's report, Spivak proudly reviewed the "thoroughly democratic" work of the JCRS, located in the "open" American West. He reported that the institution had treated close to 2,000 patients by 1913, about 30 percent of whom had entered as emergency cases. In treating patients in extremis, the JCRS was one of the few sanatoriums in the nation that admitted patients beyond the incipient or moderate stage. This policy was largely a result of Spivak's view, radical at the time, which held that patients in all stages of the disease deserved treatment. A lover of statistics, Spivak reported that 71 percent of the patients hailed from Russia, and the largest percentage had been involved in the needle trades.[2] Although the vast majority of patients at the early JCRS were Jewish, small numbers of gentiles were admitted from the beginning. Spivak was a proponent of this policy. The minutes of a JCRS Executive Committee meeting held in April 1911 reveal that he favored admitting non-Jewish patients in recognition of the modest financial support for the sanatorium contributed from the general community.[3]

Spivak's reputation within the Denver Jewish community, as a writer as well as a physician, propelled him into an innovative venture in 1915. His highly readable and eclectic writing style enabled Spivak to move with ease from technical medical writing to works designed for a popular audience. One of his best-received projects was the creation in 1915 of a new local community-wide Jewish newspaper, *The Denver Jewish News*, which for several years showcased Spivak's fresh and lively editorials. Following the demise of the Denver *Jewish Outlook,* a periodical associated with the local German Jewish establishment, in June 1914 the new Denver Central Jewish Council had considered the idea of a new local Jewish newspaper.

Spivak had played a central role in the 1912 creation of the council, a federated Jewish community umbrella association. In fact, it was Spivak who suggested the council's original motto, taken from *Proverbs*: "In a multitude of counsel there is wisdom." The council's membership was composed of two delegates from each of Denver's thirty-four Jewish organizations, including synagogues, the two Jewish hospital/sanatoriums, and various Jewish philanthropic and social groups. Spivak's close friend Rabbi Charles Kauvar, spiritual leader of the traditional Beth HaMedrosh Hagodol (BMH) Synagogue, was elected president of the new organization for a three-year term.[4]

As a member of the council committee appointed to explore the idea of a new paper, Spivak's active imagination rolled into gear. Nearly four decades after Charles Spivak had helped found *The Denver Jewish News,* his widow, Jennie Charsky Spivak, humorously recalled its origins. According to Jennie, after several weeks at work on the project, Spivak arrived home in an excited state, announcing, "I have the paper all set up, ready to print, but I have no name for it. I'll wash dishes and sweep for a whole week, if you will name this new baby of mine." Jennie reported that a bargain was concluded, and *The Denver Jewish News* appeared on the scene a few weeks later. Spivak enlisted his energetic teenage daughter Deena to serve as the salesperson, paying her to approach local doctors who were Spivak's friends to sign up for subscriptions. "I gave her fifty cents to start booming my paper. She'll get subscribers, I am sure. She has great persuasive power," he reportedly said. Spivak served as the first editor of the paper, which initially charged one dollar a year for a subscription, and he contributed many articles in his typical entertaining and informative style.[5]

In his popular writings, Spivak continued to be a champion of his fellow East European Jewish immigrants. In one of his liveliest articles in *The Denver Jewish News*, he referred to the Russian Jews who populated Denver's west side neighborhood as "the aristocrats among the Denver Jews." There, he maintained, charity might be collected and dispersed along "old-fashioned lines," but it would be "given whole-heartedly." He also asserted that "more money and brains are spent on Jewish education [in Colfax] than in all other districts of Denver put together," an area that featured both traditional Orthodox Jewish synagogues and schools and more radical socialist Jewish institutions that emphasized secular Jewish culture and nationalism.[6]

Despite Spivak's obvious appreciation and affection for the more observant west side Jews, his often contradictory outlook was also evident in his support of both the traditional Jewish practice of the use of the *mikvah* (ritual bath) by married women at the end of the menstrual cycle (which many Americanized Jews at the time considered outmoded) and his advocacy of autopsy as an aid to medical and scientific knowledge, a practice generally forbidden by traditional *halacha*, or Jewish law. In Spivak's article "Post Mortem Examinations among the Jews," published in *The New York Journal of Medicine*, he admitted that Jewish tradition did not allow the practice unless it would *directly* help save another life.

Nevertheless, in the essay, which was reprinted in Jewish periodicals all over the country, Spivak urged Jewish physicians to press for a change based on his belief that in certain cases, autopsies would provide research helpful to ultimately save lives in the future.[7] However, despite his call for "reform" of Jewish autopsy practice, Spivak generally defended Orthodox Jewish practices, such as the dietary laws of *kashrut*, in part because he believed they encouraged a healthy diet and purer ingredients, essential in particular for tuberculosis victims. Spivak's East Coast friend and colleague, fellow immigrant Dr. Maurice Fishberg, who served as the medical examiner for New York City's United Hebrew Charities, adhered to a similar outlook.[8]

Spivak's breadth of knowledge of literature and history as well as Jewish sources informed much of his writing, as in the case of a front-page editorial that appeared in *The Denver Jewish News* in January 1916 titled "Why Jews Are Not Prohibitionists." He began by documenting the disproportionate Jewish participation in reform movements but asserted that "the prohibition movement is alone an exception to the above rule." He was quick to point out that while the incidence of alcoholism was rare among Jews at the time, they "cannot and will not be prohibitionists" because their appreciation for wine was connected to Jewish spiritualism and the sanctification of Jewish customs. His knowledgeable reliance on Jewish biblical sources made the editorial especially appealing to the newspaper's readers, who would have approvingly agreed with his summation "[i]nstead of the expression, 'Come and let us have a drink,' the Jews says: 'Come and let us "make brocho" [blessing], pronounce a benediction.' "[9]

Although Spivak's writing style was generally benign, if somewhat wry, he reacted vehemently and critically to a proposal by a local Milwaukee rabbi who had called for an "effort on behalf of true Americanism to wean folk away from Yiddish." In a *Denver Jewish News* editorial provocatively titled "Rabbi Hirschberg He Does Not Like Yiddish," Spivak took the Milwaukee leader to task. Spivak's affection and respect for the Yiddish language had long occupied a central role in his life. As a champion of the East European cultural heritage, Spivak pointed out that some of the most respected works of contemporary Jewish literature had been translated into English, and those who spoke Yiddish were among the most cultured and sensitive individuals. Spivak's pen dripped with sarcasm as he advised Hirschberg that "[a] man who writes such a wooden English as the reverend gentleman does, should not rush into print and give opinions about matters he does not know the very *alef beth* [abc's]." Spivak's biting conclusion reflected the antagonisms that still surfaced at times between the older established Jewish community and the East European immigrants, with whom Spivak most closely identified. The usually mild and tolerant Spivak was moved to rail: "He [Hirschberg] does not know Yiddish. He does not know the psychology of a people and his love for his language. He does not know what liberty means. He is not a true patriot, either in the American or in the Jewish sense, and he certainly does not know what he is talking about."[10]

Throughout the period during which Spivak served as editor of *The Denver Jewish News*, he not only continued his work at the JCRS and treated private patients but also carried on medical research and writing. One of Spivak's most unusual investigations was his study of the weight of different body parts. According to a list of his writings that was published after his death, Spivak authored two articles on the topic: one titled "The Specific Gravity of the Human Body," which appeared in the April 1915 issue of *Archives of Internal Medicine,* and a second piece that focused on "Methods of Weighing Parts of the Living Human Body," which appeared later the same year in the *Journal of the American Medical Association*.[11]

Always creative, Spivak's methodology for the gravity project, according to family lore, was to place a large tank of water on his back porch and induce local newsboys to take part in the experiment by paying them fifty cents. The newsboy would submerge a limb in the tank, the displaced water would then be measured, and from this rather curious procedure the weight of the body part was calculated.[12] Spivak was still developing his ideas on the subject years later. A letter from a mechanical engineer in 1921 indicates that Spivak had consulted the man for advice on several projects, including the gravity experiment. "That other proposition of yours in getting the specific gravity of various parts of the human body was good if nothing more than it introduced some people to water," Alfred Pick noted tongue-in-cheek.[13]

The topic of Jews and medicine especially interested Spivak, and one article he authored on the subject later found its way into *The Denver Jewish News*. The typescript of the essay "The Jewish Physicians of Colorado," located in Spivak's personal collection, chronicled the lives and contributions of three of Colorado's first Jewish doctors and quantified the articles written by forty-five of his Jewish contemporary physicians in the state. According to Spivak's meticulous research, from 1871 to 1921 Colorado Jewish doctors had published a total of 4,747 medical articles. The latter statistics may have formed the basis of the article "Contributions of Colorado Jewish Physicians to Medical Literature," published in *The Denver Jewish News* in 1924.[14]

Soon after he became *The Denver Jewish News* editor, Spivak cemented his place in the larger American Jewish community when he traveled over 2,000 miles round-trip to Chicago to attend a one-day conference that resulted in the formation of the Jewish National Committee on Tuberculosis. Called together by Spivak's friend Dr. Boris Bogen, the field secretary of the National Conference of Jewish Charities, Spivak was one of twelve delegates who converged in Chicago from Denver, Cincinnati, Detroit, and New York. The group's goal was to adopt a method to register Jewish tuberculosis victims throughout the country and to unify and standardize admissions to the two national Jewish tuberculosis institutions in Denver, the NJH and the JCRS. According to Spivak, "This conference wrote a new page in the history of the crusade against tuberculosis. . . . The problem of tuberculosis among Jews has been declared by the Committee to be a *national* problem." Spivak made the motion to establish a registration bureau, which was seconded by Chicago's noted social worker Minnie Low, nicknamed the "Jane Addams of the Jews" and president of the National Council of Jewish Charities. Spivak and Low were appointed to serve on a committee "to arrange the method and proper machinery for the registration."[15]

The egalitarian spirit of the American West provided the ideal backdrop in which to nurture Spivak's eclectic talents and liberal outlook. As a transplanted westerner, Spivak surely felt in at least a psychological sense that he had "come home." While some historians have maintained that the region's celebratory liberalism and openness was largely a myth, for Spivak, compared to restrictive life in Russia, the possibilities for individual expression and the creation of meaningful social welfare institutions in America were very real. Life in Denver validated his belief in democratic socialism and his evolving commitment to American-style democracy. Although for many years the majority of JCRS patients were "Russian" Jews, as early as 1914 Spivak proudly reported diversity within that patient population: "We have in our institution Chasidim [Orthodox Jews] and agnostics, Jews and

Christians, republicans and progressives, socialists and anarchists, men of all kinds of religious, political, and economic opinions."[16] A few years after Spivak's death in 1927, Dr. Hillkowitz observed: "That indefinable feeling of freedom, satisfaction and democracy, which pervades the Institution [the JCRS] and which [is] summed up in the words of 'JCRS Spirit,' has been generated all these years by Dr. Spivak in his position as executive officer of the Society. This priceless heritage we shall endeavor to preserve intact."[17]

Nearly a decade after the JCRS opened, it was still providing free care to all patients. Most were in dire financial straits, as Spivak testified: "Ninety per cent of the patients come here penniless. It is enough to state that not 5% of our patients come here at their own expense. Whatever money they bring with them, which is, as a rule, very little, they spend here for their board while waiting. When they enter the Sanatorium their purses are empty and consequently when the time comes to leave the Sanatorium they find themselves in a sore predicament. The majority have not got enough money to pay for their first week's board and room."[18]

As the years passed, one evident physical change on the sanatorium campus was that the distinctive tent-cottages that had characterized the early JCRS had given way to a significant extent to buildings with patient wards. In his superintendent's report for 1913, Dr. Herman Schwatt (who was Spivak's brother-in-law) called the tents "[a] survival of that mistaken idea in treatment of tuberculosis—the idea of the so-called 'roughing it' treatment. . . . I hope that the time is not far distant in the future when all our patients will be housed in properly constructed buildings."[19] Dr. Spivak later echoed Schwatt's sentiments when calling for additional buildings to house patients. He purported that "instead of a help to the patients, they [the tents] are a menace to them," reflecting his evolving views on what constituted the best environment for tuberculosis patients. His words also reveal Spivak's willingness to change his mind when presented with compelling evidence. In the summer the tents proved too hot to enable the patients to rest comfortably, and in the winter, even with additional blankets, the tents were often too cold to sleep in.[20]

Over the years, Spivak's imprint continued to be most clearly felt in the sanatorium's homelike atmosphere, as the JCRS closely resembled the late-nineteenth- and early-twentieth-century hospital, which had not yet begun its development toward the "modern" Progressive-Era complex. As was true of many nineteenth-century community hospitals, the JCRS was more like a private home or a small hotel rather than the formal hospital setting we know today.[21] What is perhaps most unique about the JCRS is that this atmosphere persisted so far into the twentieth century, even as late as the Great Depression of the 1930s. Moreover, while most hospitals of the era were controlled by upper-middle-class trustees, who for decades had exerted total control over even mundane matters,[22] at the JCRS three doctors—Spivak, Hillkowitz, and Zederbaum—were undoubtedly the most powerful figures among the trustees. This reflected both the strength of their personalities and perhaps the general high regard in which physicians were held historically by Jews. In Europe, medicine had been one of the few respected professional fields Jews were allowed to enter. Jewish immigrants brought a tradition of high value placed on health care with them to the United States. Initially in Europe and then later in America, a doctor was most often greeted in a Jewish home with respect and awe. Even Orthodox Jewish rabbis emphasized that a physician could be called whenever necessary, as a doctor was "God's instrument in healing the sick," and health was essential to carrying out God's commandments.[23]

Nationally recognized social worker Chester Teller was highly impressed with the atmosphere at the JCRS. In a report published in 1916 he observed, "The relations between officers and patients is [sic] informal and sympathetic. The patients, or guests as they are sometimes spoken of, constitute a kind of big family . . . a spirit of camaraderie and fellowship pervades the place."[24] While the tone at the JCRS was warm, the strict rules were not without critics, as tuberculosis patients who felt ill could easily become agitated. For the most part, however, those who "chased the cure" at the JCRS would have agreed with the observations of patient Louis Gross, who had been admitted to several sanatoriums before landing at the JCRS. He was especially critical of another experience in which "I was in a sanatorium supported entirely by Jewish charity funds, yet I found not a modicum of Judaism there." He went on to describe his arrival at "beloved Dr. Spivak's hotel," nothing the kosher food and the Jewish and personal ambiance at the JCRS.[25]

At the helm of the JCRS, Spivak continued to assist immigrant Jewish patients in maintaining their ethnic and religious traditions by providing a comfort zone as they made the transition to becoming Americans. Spivak, a voracious reader, felt that books and magazines would divert patients' attention from a fixation on their illness and "take them out of themselves."[26] However, reading and educational lectures were supplemented by classes in spelling and writing the English language for East European immigrant patients. In this way, although the JCRS was dedicated to perpetuating Jewish culture among the patients, it also fostered Americanization. Physicians and ethnic-based hospitals of the period often served as "significant cultural mediators" as new immigrants who arrived during the mass migration of the late nineteenth and early twentieth centuries were integrated into American society.[27]

Having arrived in the United States in 1882 during what historians have termed the "long century" of immigration, Spivak clearly understood the importance of acquiring English skills as an essential tool in his upward mobility. Spivak began life in the United States as a laborer, but once he had acquired a good command of English he was able to move into a respected profession, a trajectory he undoubtedly hoped many of his patients would follow. Surely, Spivak and the JCRS as a whole served as successful and primary agents in the acculturation process for many East European Jews.

Spivak put his talent for writing and his English skills to good use working on JCRS publications. Spivak had written for the institution's official periodical, *The Sanatorium*, from its inception. He formally became the editor in 1911, replacing his good friend Dr. Philip Hillkowitz, who had shepherded the publication during its first few years. According to the JCRS minutes of July 19, 1911, Spivak reported that he had offered his services as editor because "he considers the publication as one of the best means of propaganda that the J.C.R.S. has." In a reference to his modest income, Spivak maintained that "if he could afford it he would have taken the work without remuneration." The minutes reveal that Spivak was to be paid $1,500 a year, approved unanimously by a secret ballot among the board members present.[28]

It is apparent that Spivak especially enjoyed collecting and disseminating data. In addition to his often pithy editorials in *The Sanatorium*, he carefully compiled patient statistics that still provide researchers with valuable demographic profiles of thousands of men and women who were treated at the institution. These rich sources included information on nativity, occupation, duration of disease, and ethnic and religious origin. Over the years, Dr. Spivak continued to fill the pages of *The Sanatorium* with useful information. In 1924, for example, he published an important report on "The Mortality of the Jews in Denver," a careful study of the main causes of death for Denver's Jewish citizens from 1900 to 1920.[29]

Far from a dry source of facts and numbers and public relations solicitations, *The Sanatorium* clearly reflected Spivak's literate yet humorous and engaging style, filled as it was with history, medical lore, and dramatic human interest stories. Additionally, the publication made others outside Denver's Jewish community aware of his writing talent. When the Colorado Medical Society published a commemorative volume, *Medical Coloradoana*, on its fiftieth anniversary in 1921, the society's leaders turned to Spivak, who compiled the extensive lists of published articles by Colorado physicians. Spivak was also the author of an important article on the "History of Medicine in the Bible and Talmud" and another essay on Jewish physicians that appeared in *The Jewish Encyclopedia* in 1901 (reprinted in the 1916 and 1925 editions). In his writings, Spivak often pointed out the great respect Jewish tradition placed on medicine and used the famous dictum from the Talmud (Sanhedrin 17b) that "it is forbidden to live in a city without a physician" to prove his point.[30]

Sometime around 1917, during the second decade of the JCRS, the U.S. tuberculosis movement reached maturity, and the Denver sanatorium continued to focus on areas that preoccupied the national crusade. In addition to the daily treatment regimen supervised by the medical superintendent, under Spivak's guidance the JCRS continued to emphasize mass public education about the disease. This was accomplished through public lectures and the institution's publications, and the JCRS administration cooperated with health professionals and institutions throughout the country to raise awareness. *The Sanatorium* featured regular articles about the causes, prevention, and treatment of the disease authored by leading experts, and Dr. Spivak lectured widely on health and hygiene issues.

Spivak's continuing involvement in the national tuberculosis movement was evidenced in a short article titled "Meeting the Problem of the Indigent Tuberculous among the Jews," which he published in a 1919 issue of the JCRS *Sanatorium*. Expanding the emphasis on coordinating tuberculosis treatment within the American Jewish community, initiated a few years earlier at the Chicago meeting, Spivak observed that many tuberculosis victims were poor to begin with. They then became dependent as the disease robbed them of both their limited financial resources and their means of making a living. He suggested a dual approach to meet the problem. First, Spivak called for expanded fundraising to support both the institutions that provided medical treatment for the ill and their families. Second, he urged local and national registration of those afflicted with tuberculosis, including those already being treated in sanatoriums or hospitals, and yearly exams for adults and children throughout the country to provide early diagnosis of tuberculosis.[31] This latter notion became a central tenet in the national tuberculosis campaign.

Long hours engaged in administrative and medical work at the JCRS ate into the time Charles Spivak could spend on his private medical practice, which frequently left the Spivak family in strained circumstances. After eight years of totally voluntary service to the sanatorium, Spivak was persuaded to accept a modest salary. According to one report, in 1916 Spivak's salary was listed as $3,500.[32] A colleague later declared that for the sake of the JCRS, Spivak "left his lucrative medical practice and gave up his professorial chair at the University to take charge of the affairs of the sanatorium."[33]

Throughout his long career, Spivak's wife and children continued to be the anchors of his life. Spivak's views on the centrality of family are vividly revealed in a 1907 letter he wrote to Dr. Michael Ball on the occasion of the birth of his friend's first child. Enthusiastically wishing Ball "a thousand congratulations," Spivak reminded Ball that he had long predicted "this bliss which you were wanting" and that "supreme happiness can come to you only through them [wife and children]." He applauded Ball's choice of a biblical name for his daughter. "I like biblical names," Spivak wrote. "All my children are thus named."[34]

Despite challenges and sometimes dashed expectations, Spivak remained a doting father and loyal husband throughout his life. His eldest daughter, Deena Spivak Strauss, recalled that notwithstanding his busy schedule, Dr. Spivak made it a point to be home for dinner each night so he could interact with his wife and children. Yet from the family's perspective, the time he spent with them was only "adequate." Still, he took a keen interest in their daily challenges and triumphs, and dinner conversation was never dull with the garrulous Jenny, Charles, Deena, and Ruth at the table. Son David, nicknamed "Doodie," was considered more reserved.[35]

Spivak's familiarity with all forms of literature helped make his conversation and letters enjoyable. Deena observed that her father was an avid reader and that the family dining room table was seldom used for meals because it was covered with books, magazines, and newspapers. According to Deena, Dr. Spivak often stood over the cleaning lady while she worked in the room to make sure none of his materials were moved. His speeches and conversation were so interesting, she declared, because they were always interwoven with bits of a poem, a quote from an engaging piece of literature, or commentary on current events.[36] Spivak read widely, and he often ordered volumes from booksellers in New York City. In one letter Spivak notified a dealer that he was enclosing a check for "Rappaport's book" for $1.65 but did not care to pay $1.50 for a copy of Dostoyevsky's *Fathers and Sons.* "If however, you come across a second-hand copy cheap, bound or unbound, you may send it to me," he instructed.[37]

Spivak's familiarity with literature classics was evident in an editorial in a 1911 issue of the JCRS *Sanatorium* in which he reviewed "The Consumptive in Literature." "All the great writers of the last century have made good use of the consumptive," wrote Spivak and proceeded to cite Dumas's drama *Dame aux Camille* (later made into the popular film *Camille*) and Shaw's play *The Doctor's Dilemma,* as well as works by Balzac, Tolstoy, Chekoff [sic], and numerous Yiddish writers. The piece was meant to introduce a regular fictional feature in future issues of *The Sanatorium* that would highlight the plight of tuberculosis victims and encourage patients to develop their literary horizons.[38] Spivak later encouraged JCRS patients to compile their own publications. The *Tales of the Tents*, edited by patients, appeared in 1914 but was curtailed in 1917 for financial reasons. However, Spivak proudly congratulated the editors of the revived periodical, named *Hatikvah* (Hope), when it made its debut in 1923 featuring poems, short stories, and practical advice for tuberculosis victims.[39]

Unlike many men and women who made broad "humanity" alone the object of their compassion and concern, Spivak's devotion certainly extended to his own family. All too often, successful men of the era were neglectful of family and friends, as in the case of Spivak's fellow immigrant physician Dr. Joseph Goldberger, who discovered the cure for pellagra.[40] When Deena was a small child in grammar school, she was greeted at the end of a snowy day by her father, who carried her home because he was afraid she would become distressed or even lost in the snowstorm. Dr.

Spivak's office was located in a set of rooms in the Court Street house, and as a child the talkative Deena liked to visit with his patients in the waiting room, offering a combination of medical and personal "advice." She recalled one day when Spivak scolded her, although with a characteristic twinkle in his eye, and tartly requested she leave the premises so he could "tend to my own patients."[41]

In an era when letter writing was the primary mode of communication, Spivak family members were energetic and lively practitioners of the art. Charles Spivak's personal files contain scores of letters and several school essays written by his daughters Deena and Ruth and son David that were precious enough for him to save for decades. David's artwork was displayed with pride in the Spivak home, although his choice of career may have initially been somewhat of a disappointment to his workaholic father. Apparently the Spivaks' youngest child, Ruth, was an unplanned addition to the family. Six-and-a-half years younger than Deena, Ruth was often referred to fondly as "the accident" by her mother, Jennie.[42]

In June 1915 Charles Spivak took a trip to San Francisco, California, to visit the Panama-Pacific International Exposition (the World's Fair) and garner support for the JCRS. Spivak's "Western Tour" was previewed in an article in *The Sanatorium*, probably written by Spivak considering the humorous tone. According to the article, "The Secretary [Spivak] had never crossed the Rocky Mountain range. He naturally wanted to see the West. He has never seen a world's fair. . . . [B]esides, he claims he needs a vacation." Spivak was to stop first in Salt Lake City and from there travel to San Francisco to make appeals at a mass meeting along with Dr. Hillkowitz, followed by appearances in San Diego and Los Angeles.[43]

The Panama-Pacific International Exposition opened in February 1915 in San Francisco to celebrate the completion of the Panama Canal and, more likely, to demonstrate the city's impressive recovery after the devastating 1906 earthquake. Given Spivak's eclectic interests and passion for science, he was undoubtedly fascinated by the impressive sights including a "gem"-covered Tower of Jewels, the Palace of Fine Arts, the Palace of Horticulture, and the Avenue of Nations. On June 22, 1915, an earthquake struck California's Imperial Valley, and Spivak's daughters immediately wrote him two anxious letters. First Deena and then Ruth expressed their concern. "Today makes the third day that we haven't received any word from you," Deena chided in a typed letter. She continued:

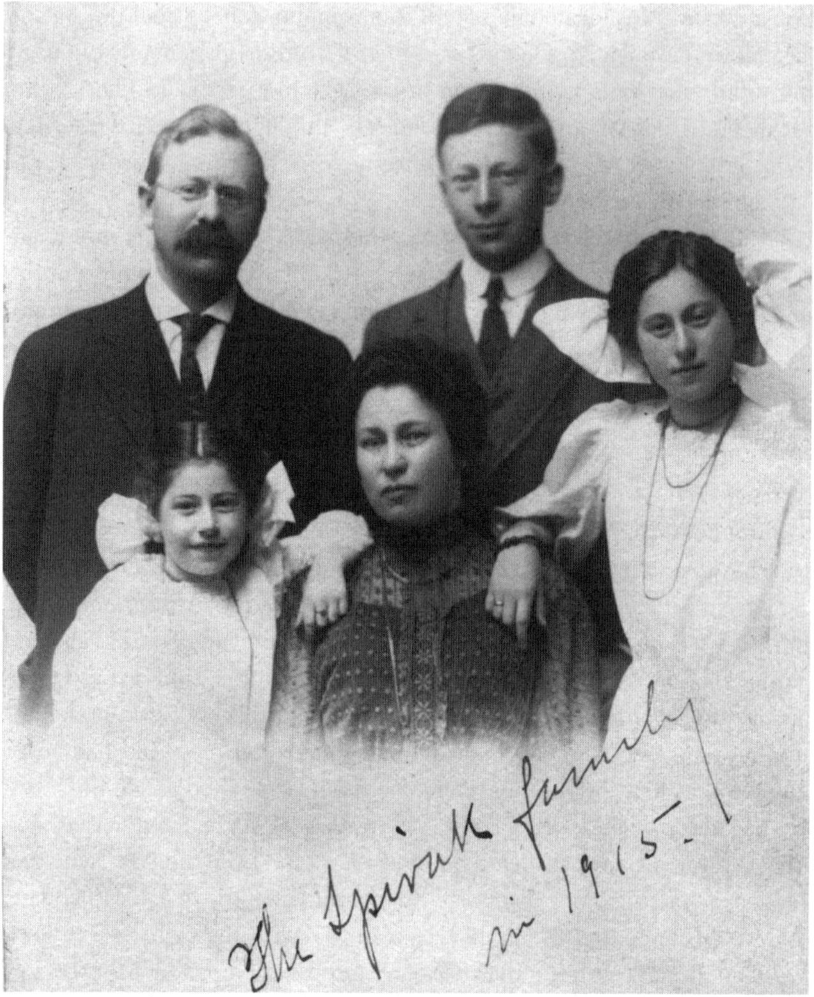

The Spivak family in 1915. Standing (left to right): Dr. Charles David Spivak, David Spivak, Deena Spivak. Seated (left to right): Ruth Spivak, Jennie Charsky Spivak. Courtesy, Charlesa Wolfe Feinstein.

Why is it that you do not write? Surely you could spare five minutes of your time to drop us a postal, couldn't you? I am using some of your own arguments, you see. If it weren't for the earthquake we wouldn't worry . . . but papa dear, the suspense is terrible. Of course I know you aren't in the quake zone yet, but you are going there. . . . For my part, there is nothing that I would like better than to see, and feel, the quake,

> but for you I am afraid. I know you are perfectly able to take care of yourself, and others too, but still I am afraid. Do stay away from that vicinity, won't you? You have seen the fair by now, what is it like? Does it come up to your expectations? Do tell us all about it, don't wait until you get home.[44]

Unfortunately, Dr. Spivak's own description of the World's Fair does not appear in the correspondence. The next day Ruth, then age fourteen, added her exhortations: "What is the reason you do not write? I have not studied my lessons yet so I cannot write much. Papa, please do not go near the earthquake zone. We are all worried about you. I have about one million questions to ask you when you get home. Don't forget our Middies and mamma's Ring. . . . Mamma walked out to the city park museum and back again today, just for the fun of it. Your loving Ruth."[45]

Dr. Spivak returned safely to Colorado and back to work at the JCRS with additional funding for the sanatorium in his pocket. By August 1915 Deena and Ruth were vacationing in the state's famous hot springs resort at Idaho Springs, located in the foothills of the Rocky Mountains about thirty-five miles west of Denver. Ruth's note to her parents thanks them for their many letters and in particular for the money sent by Dr. Spivak. After a brisk morning of tennis, Ruth reported that "[w]e are having the time of our lives up here . . . all we do up here is eat. The town is about as big as a yawn. I love the water of the hot springs." Deena added her remarks in a separate letter: "How do you like the car? Have you gotten it yet? Mamma dear, do you suppose you would be able to send us up some stuff for a lunch. We want to take our lunch up in the hills Friday, but it costs so much here . . . and really we can't afford it."[46]

The entire Spivak family was involved with the work of the JCRS, and Dr. Spivak obviously made a concerted effort to ensure they were included from the beginning, when Jennie was brought on as a formal JCRS incorporator. For many years Deena, Ruth, and Jennie were associated with plays or theatricals performed at the sanatorium for the benefit of the patients and patrons, serving variously as actors or authors as the situation warranted. Deena authored one play called *The Spirit of the JCRS,* which starred Ruth and was performed in Dallas, Texas, as a fundraiser for the sanatorium.[47] Ruth especially had an interest in drama and delivering recitations, and in the 1923 *Denver City Directory* her occupation was listed as actress and in 1927 as "dramatic arts."[48] She taught dancing, drama, and elocution and later married Dr. Joseph Wolfe of Dallas. Ruth became very active in small theater work there. The couple became the parents of two children, daughter Charlesa, named in memory of Dr. Spivak, and son David, named after Ruth's brother.

Field secretaries for the sanatorium were a highly varied group, and one of the most interesting JCRS representatives was Deena Spivak, who was enrolled at the University of Colorado in Boulder before she took a leave of absence to work for the JCRS. Apparently her decision to attend college in Boulder may have initially been a source of dissension in the family, and there was some concern over her prospects for academic success, as in an early letter to her father she felt compelled to offer an apology. "I'm so sorry, papa dear," Deena wrote, "that I have been the cause of so much strife in our family. Never mind dear, we'll just show them (1) that you and I were right in going to Boulder (2nd) that I am not going to flunk."[49]

From Deena's remarks, it appears that Dr. Spivak championed his elder daughter's enrollment in college, particularly at a college not located in her hometown, although Boulder was only about thirty-five miles from Denver. As we have seen, when he helped facilitate his wife's college career, Charles Spivak was ahead of his time in support of higher education for women, and his encouragement extended to his daughter as well. Deena moved to Boulder in August 1915, renting a room for eight dollars a week and settling for secondhand books because of the high cost of new ones. Jennie was in New York City with her son, David, at the time, as Deena asked whether Spivak and Ruth had heard from her yet.[50]

By the next month, Deena had settled into the college routine, and Jennie Spivak was still in New York. "Don't forget folks that the sixth of October is Mama's birthday. I think we ought to send her something nice, don't you?" she instructed her father and sister. She also recommended that "Baby" Ruth, as she affectionately called her younger sister, "take it easy" and get plenty of sleep so she could pay adequate attention in school. Deena, who gave private piano lessons to children in Boulder, was determined to make a career out of music and singing. She was understandably disappointed that she "did not make the choir. . . . What makes me sorriest of all is that I know that I sing much better than either of the two altos that were chosen." Deena, rarely short of confidence, consoled herself that "it is not a matter of voice, it[']s pull, up here. Don't think, however, that I am discouraged. No indeed, if I'm here next year, I'll try out again; I'm not boasting when I tell you I sing better, it is a fact."[51] Winter brought cold weather, and she soon wrote to ask Dr. Spivak to send her "something" to treat her sore throat and fever. She related, "We had a perfectly good exam in Algebra. Yes I did it full justice." Deena also reported, "Got a letter from Mamma. She didn't say much except that she was lonesome. Poor little kiddie. Well, I'm glad that she has Doodie [son David] at least."[52]

In December 1915 Deena wrote her father from Boulder:

> I got your rebuke [about not writing] this morning. . . . I'm sorry that I wasn't able to come in [to Denver] last Friday. . . . I sang at the Young Woman's Christian Assoc. the other day. Of course, I don't know how it sounded, but [my friend] Gladys told me she had never heard me sing so well. . . . Now you see with raising my grades and taking part in girls' affairs, I don't have much time for "fussing." I got my six weeks grades yesterday. . . . I feel very proud of myself. . . . I'm so glad that Baby [Ruth] is in such demand. It is the best thing in the world for her. It will give her confidence in herself. That's what she needs.[53]

Although the reference to Ruth being in "demand" is unclear, it was likely related to dramatic recitations she performed at the JCRS, at school, or for small public audiences.

At age twenty-one, Deena Spivak left school for a period between 1916 and 1917 and toured countless small southern and midwestern towns spreading the JCRS "message." A speech Deena delivered in St. Louis resulted in funding for the landmark JCRS water tower. Dr. Spivak frequently sent Deena checks to cover her traveling expenses, and in one postcard she thanked him for the money and complained "[y]ou have no idea what the expenses are here! To go from Richmond to Norfolk takes four and a half hours and they charge six dollars. Awful!"[54] A letter dated December 4, 1916, from Deena to her father recounted a hectic schedule filled with luncheons, dinners, and theatrical entertainments shared with southern Jews who were potential supporters. At the end of the letter Deena concluded, "In between times I gather in subscriptions with different people."[55]

An attractive, articulate, and vivacious young woman, Deena managed to collect not only funds but also marriage proposals as she traveled the country.[56] In a letter to her family from Charleston, South Carolina, written in January 1917, she informed her parents and sister that she had sent a box of letters home, presumably from her admirers, and she cautioned the family to "[p]lease do me a favor, *don't read any of them.*"[57] In another letter Deena penned an affectionate note to her father from Norfolk, Virginia, on the occasion of his fifty-fifth birthday. Deena was in the South at the time raising funds. "May you live to be a hundred and fifty-five," she wrote and added a sentence in Yiddish wishing him "gesunt um glicklich" (health and joy).[58]

Upon her return, Deena completed her studies at the University of Colorado (CU) in Boulder, majoring in literature. While still a student she married Herman Strauss, a former engineering student at CU who had returned to teach at his alma mater. Strauss was captivated by Deena's vivid, bold personality. Herman and Deena started their married life in Boulder, but they moved to Denver after the birth of their first child. Herman later became a successful entrepreneur in the floor products business. The couple became the parents of "three and a half children," as Deena put it. A boy and two girls were born to the Strausses: Donald Strauss, Adele Strauss Karsh, and Ruth Strauss Oppenheim. Later, in the 1930s, they took in a foster son named Carl, a German Jewish Holocaust refugee.[59] Dr. Spivak doted on his grandchildren. According to one source, he was frequently seen on the JCRS grounds pushing Deena's daughter Adele around in her buggy, bouncing the carriage up and down to make the baby laugh.[60]

Jennie and Charles's eldest child, David, who had been born on November 19, 1893, in Philadelphia, was attracted to art from a young age. Educated in Denver elementary schools, he graduated from South High School, where he played football. After high school, David Spivak enrolled briefly at the University of Denver, where his mother, Jennie, taught Russian, before moving on to Chicago's famed Art Institute. In the 1912 *Denver City Directory* he is listed as a "student."[61]

After a few years David left for New York City to spend three years studying at the Art Students League under respected artist and teacher Robert Henri. His sister Deena recalled that both Charles and Jennie Spivak felt David had serious artistic talent that needed to be nurtured. Jennie accompanied David to New York City for what was intended to be a three-week visit while she helped him set up an apartment, but apparently she stayed for quite awhile. With Deena in college in Boulder and David and Jennie in New York, Ruth was left at home with her father so she could attend high school.

While the family was close, fragments of family letters hint at some strife over David's choice of career in the early years, and at least one of Spivak's friends saw David as less than a success. It is likely that the artistically inclined Jennie was supportive of David's career choice while Charles Spivak was either ambivalent or impatient with his son as he tried to "find" himself. While Spivak evidently supported his daughters in their artistic endeavors and in women's right to higher education in general, it appears he may have set the bar higher for his only son, perhaps hoping he would follow him into medicine. In the 1920s, on a trip to New York City, Spivak ran into his old friend Dr. Michael Ball, who noted the event in his diary. "I met [journalist Abraham] Cahan several times. I saw Spivak, the first time in years, when he visited New York, and I met his son, David, whose Godfather I am. David has tried art and newspaper work, but he has failed in most things."[62] The "newspaper work" Ball referred to was probably graphic art illustrations.

Several letters from David to Charles and Ruth Spivak, written in 1915, demonstrate that all was not harmonious between David and Charles at the time. "It is impossible for me to understand the attitude you have taken in answering my letters," wrote David bitterly, and he also hints at "trouble" his father might be experiencing. "By that I mean not answering them at all. . . . If you are no longer interested in what I do or what I say, why I will not write at all. . . . I started in Moran's Life Class last Monday as I thought I needed criticism and practice. . . . I will have to close as ma is anxious to get to the Specktorsky's early tonight." The letter is signed "Your loving son, Doodie."[63]

However, things may have been smoothed over, for the next month David wrote a cheerful and encouraging letter to his "baby" sister Ruth, advising her to find a friend with whom she could get some exercise, particularly as a skating partner. He also reported he was sorry to learn that she had stopped her daily elocution lessons, as "every one says you recite so well." David revealed the great joy he received from his artwork, noting, "after you have finished your creation, after you have had all the pleasure yourself, there it is for whoever looks at it to find pleasure and enjoyment too. Well can you beat that? Of course all the arts are the same in that respect only painting has them all beat." He concluded, "Everything is about the same here. It seems as if every one has forsaken you. . . . Mother, brother and sister have all left only papa is there to fill the awful gaps. It will be a comfort to you to know that ma is feeling fine and that the change has done her a lot of good. P.S. I wanted to say something cheerful but it came out the other way. Personally, I think we are a very lucky and happy family and have absolutely nothing to pity ourselves about."[64]

A letter Jennie Spivak wrote to Ruth while she was in New York also gives insight into both the family dynamics and Jennie's rather high-strung, emotional style. Several letters allude to Jennie's health but do not spell out whether she was suffering from a respiratory relapse or a form of nervous exhaustion. Written toward the end of the school year, the letter is addressed to "Dearest sweetest Rissele" (the Yiddish affectionate diminutive of Ruth). Jennie implored Ruth to join her in New York with its many attractions, including the ocean and the Metropolitan Museum. Perhaps trying to convince Ruth by prompting feelings of guilt, Jennie mused as to whether her daughter had "forgotten your mamma." In an effort to influence Ruth to leave her father on his own in Denver, Jennie argued, "Papa is a full grown man, child . . . so I am sure, my sweet, he will be able to spare you for the time I am in N.Y. & let you come, & besides do not forget, my sweet, that papa has his work. . . . [Y]ou are both no company to each other, he is busy all the time, whereas, we two, my sweet child, are company & am always near you & with you; papa loves us all & I cannot see for the world of me why he would not be happy to know that we are in a place where it is best for us and he is free to arrange his work as he sees best."[65]

David experienced doubts about his ability to earn a living through his artwork, but he was exhilarated by the quest. In an undated fragment of a letter from his sister Deena that still survives, probably written while he was studying art in New York, she compliments his talent and exhorts him to persevere: "[Y]ou have plenty of that [talent] it[']s *will power* you need. Get to it Doodie. . . . Go to it, Doodie win, you can. Why don't you do it? If you have to commercialize your art for the time being, do it. . . . If there is any thing in you it won't die. Don't be a baby Doodie. Do some thing! Be *a Man*."[66]

At the same Deena, in typical, rather dramatic teenage fashion, was dreaming of making her distinct mark on the world in the field of music. She informed David that "[i]f in June Papa won't pay for my music lessons I'll work as a servant in someone's house till I get along where I can earn money for myself. Some day people are going to say the name Deena Spivak in awe. I won't stop till I get it."[67]

David Spivak's art career appears to have progressed, as he was listed as an "artist" in the 1918 *Denver City Directory*. However, with the advent of World War I, the young man was sent to Kelly Field in Texas, where he served for a year as a member of an aviation unit. In 1919 David's residence was listed as the family home at 850 S. Franklin in the *Denver City Directory*, but there is a notation for "U.S. Army" next to his name.[68]

After World War I, David Spivak returned to Colorado, where he again turned to painting. When Dr. Spivak traveled to Poland in 1920 on a rescue mission on behalf of Jewish war refugees, the rest of the family stayed behind. An undated letter Ruth wrote to her father in Europe documents that David was still pursuing art studies at the time and receiving moral support from at least his mother and sister, as well as financial assistance from Dr. Spivak. "Dearest Papa," Ruth wrote, "Doodie [David] phoned this morning and told mama that he wired to you asking you if you would help him go to Philadelphia. Gee, I hope he can go, because he needs to see what other artists are doing around the country. . . . [W]e are all well and missing you very much."[69]

As time passed, David's work received national critical acclaim, but like the Impressionist artists he so admired, sales of his paintings never brought in enough money to support his wife and children. As time passed, the relationship between David and his father returned to being very cordial. In the summer of 1921, David and his family vacationed in the Rocky Mountains, and in July David invited his father to come and visit and bring some groceries, "if convenient," in the Spivak's automobile, or "machine" as David referred to it. "Of course if it is too much bother," David concluded, "don't trouble as I know you haven't much time and the important thing is you come up if you have the time and desire to do so. Your loving son, Doodie."[70]

As an art instructor, David Spivak taught variously in Denver at East High School, West High School, the Denver Academy of Applied Art, the Denver Institute of Art, and the Chappell School of Art. The 1923 *Denver City Directory*, for example, listed him as residing at the Spivak family home at 850 S. Franklin and his occupation as teacher.[71] By 1926 David was living with his wife, Flo (Flora), and children at 1021 Cook, but he was still listed as a teacher. The couple had three sons—Eugene, born in 1919;

Daniel, born in 1921; and David Jr., born in 1924. However, David's true avocation remained painting, and he contented himself with completing many portraits, landscapes, and murals in his "free" time. For many years a large, acclaimed mural painted by Spivak in 1927, depicting the biblical giving of the Ten Commandments on Mount Sinai, hung behind the ark of the BMH Synagogue. Several of his works are still visible in Denver today, including a large portrait of his father at the old JCRS grounds, now the Rocky Mountain College of Art and Design.

An affectionate letter David wrote to Dr. Spivak in the spring of 1925 indicated that their relationship had settled into an easy pattern. "Dear Pa," he began,

> Was surprised to hear that instead of coming you turned around and went back again. . . . How have things been coming with you on your long jaunt about the country. I hope you are not taking things too strenuously. . . . I have finished Florence's portrait and delivered same. The Radetskys seem very much pleased. . . . [Our sons] Eugene and Dan are fine. . . . Ma and Ruth are well & of course Ruth is very busy with the play. She made a deal with some fellow to handle her program & advertising on a commission basis and hopes to make about $75 from that. . . . Deena and her family all well. I see them every day. Your loving son, Doodie.[72]

By the 1920s and 1930s David Spivak had become a central figure in Denver's art community. He was a key player in the early development of the Denver Art Museum and was one of the original founders of the Denver Artists' Guild in 1928. Quoted at the opening of the guild's inaugural exhibit, David maintained that art and beauty helped make better, more humane citizens. A 1929 series of letters between David and Dr. Lee Frankel, vice president of Metropolitan Life Insurance Company in New York, indicate that David was still seeking a national reputation. Frankel, who had been born in Philadelphia, was an acknowledged pioneer in preventative health care and a longtime acquaintance of Dr. Spivak's. When Frankel stayed at the Brown Palace Hotel during a visit to Denver in 1929, David met with him and began a pastel sketch of his father's friend. He later presented it to the grateful Frankel as a gift. The letterhead on David's note reads "David Spivak, Artist." In thanking David for the "excellent likeness," Frankel remarked, "I am looking forward with interest to see-

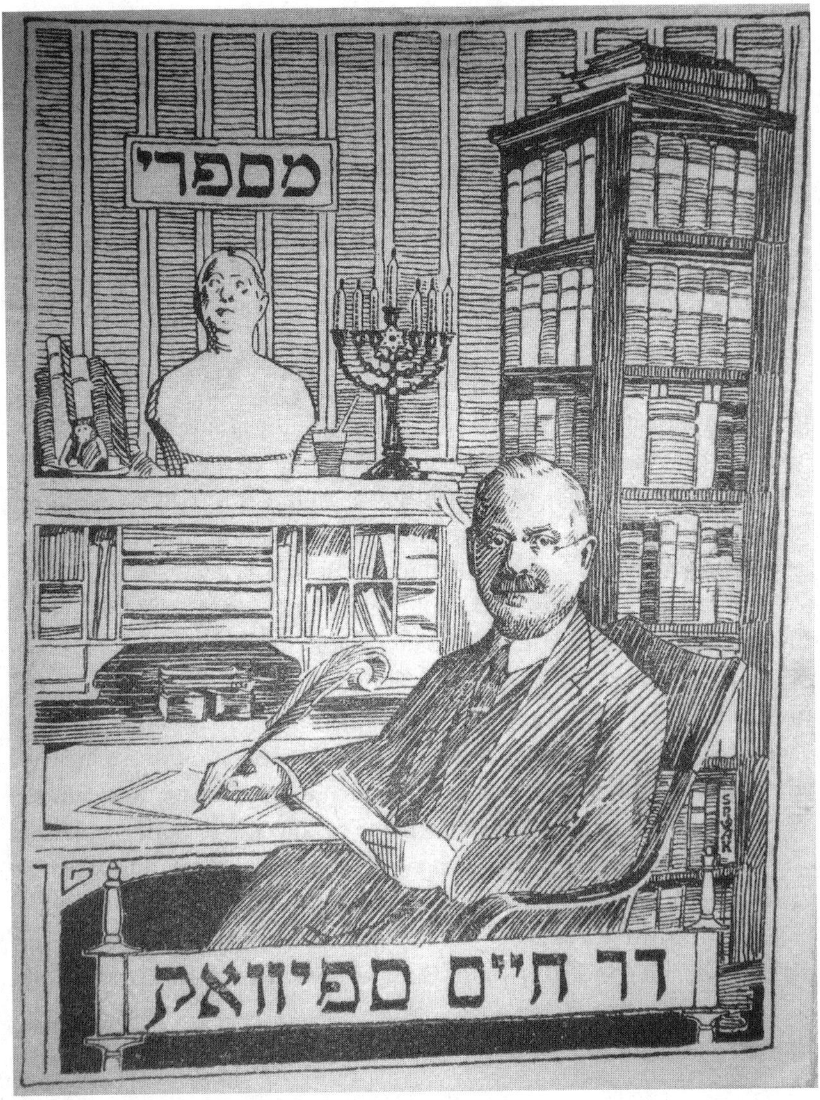

Pen-and-ink drawing of Dr. Charles David Spivak in his study by his artist son David Spivak. Courtesy, Beck Archives, Special Collections, Penrose Library, University of Denver.

ing your rapid development as an artist. The sketch which you have made indicates to my mind very clearly that you have ability and talent." He encouraged David to come to New York City, where he would have more "opportunities."[73] Sadly, David's potential was never fully realized. Just five years after the death of his father, the younger Spivak died suddenly in 1932 at age thirty-nine as the result of a brain tumor.

Shortly after David's death, the Denver Art Museum mounted an exhibit of his work. The catalog listed over 250 of his works, including portraits and landscapes painted between 1914 and 1917 and a larger group painted between 1922 and his death, which included a number of Colorado sites, several small-sized paintings of his mother, and a very large portrait of Dr. Charles Spivak that measured thirty-eight inches by fifty-three inches. A clever pen-and-ink self-portrait sketch of the artist reveals an urbane, sophisticated David Spivak smoking a pipe.[74] Spivak's work was praised in the catalog: "The Colorado sunshine, the atmosphere in relation to the Rocky Mountains, fascinated him and offered a great deal of study. When he placed the objects of his study upon the canvas, they became articulate. . . . With conciseness, clearness and conviction, each small canvas represents an artistic problem illuminated by his personal genius."[75]

While David, Deena, and Ruth Spivak matured, Dr. Spivak moved through late middle age, and his energy and dedication to what he considered his primary work—the prevention and care of tuberculosis—continued unabated. His leadership at the JCRS remained central to the organization's growth and development; and his reputation as a physician, administrator, and writer increasingly spread beyond Colorado and the West, where he had clearly made a name for himself in both the general and Jewish communities. As he approached age sixty, when many people begin to look toward a quieter life and retirement, Charles Spivak redoubled his efforts. He was always on the lookout for new projects to pursue, and a challenging trip to war-torn Europe loomed on the horizon.

7

Overseas Mission to the European Front and the Final Years

In the early 1920s Dr. Charles David Spivak took a leave of absence from the Jewish Consumptives' Relief Society (JCRS) and his private medical practice to step onto the international stage on behalf of the American Jewish community in the role of special medical commissioner to Poland through the Joint Distribution Committee (JDC). The JDC was a powerful Jewish relief agency created during World War I that aided destitute European Jews, and Spivak spent six months in war-torn Poland dispensing humanitarian assistance and collecting data about the precarious situation of Polish Jews. In the process, he also played an important part in the transference of leadership of the American Jewish community from the established German Jews to the East European newcomers and their descendants, a path foreshadowed by his key role in the formation of the JCRS.

World War I had a devastating effect on East European Jews, caught as they were in the maelstrom of conflict. Many were left homeless, food was scarce, and they were especially susceptible to epidemics such as typhus as a result of inadequate sanitation and poor nutrition. In response to the critical need, the American Jewish community organized a number of relief organizations. Most notable were the American Jewish Relief Committee, jump-started by such prominent German Jewish leaders as New York banker and philanthropist Jacob Schiff and attorney Louis Marshall, and the Orthodox Jewish–based Central Relief Committee. The Jewish working-class unions rallied around their own organization, the People's Relief Committee.

To coordinate aid among these three American Jewish charitable organizations, the American Jewish JDC, known popularly as "the Joint," was established in November 1914. The Joint's main goal was to provide and coordinate large-scale medical, financial, and social service relief to Jewish co-religionists in Europe, but it also brought German and East European Jews together in a noble cause. Money was pooled but was raised separately by each of the organizations, although the majority of the funds came from the wealthier German Jews. However, each organization was represented equally on the governing board, an unusual occurrence.

In addition to providing needed aid, the Joint also represented a critical shift in the changing of the guard in Jewish American leadership. As Arthur Hertzberg has noted, symbolically the JDC represented a turning point, for "it was the first major step forward for the East Europeans," who were increasingly wresting power from the "German Jews," who until that point had held the monopoly in the field of foreign policy. The Joint proved a crucial battle site in which, according to Hertzberg's assessment, "[t]he Russians [would] defeat the Germans," and by the early 1920s the East European immigrants and their descendants would "become the dominant force in American Jewry."[1]

The JDC received support from Herbert Hoover, administrator of the U.S. relief program in Europe, and in 1920 the U.S. State Department granted the Jewish organization permission to send a medical team to Poland to assess the situation.[2] Dr. Charles Spivak was invited to be a part of this medical field team, formally a unit of the U.S. Army, and he and his fellow physicians wore military uniforms and received their initial training and supplies in Washington, D.C. Spivak steadfastly refused to publish his memoirs, but fortunately he appeared as a supporting character in a number of reminiscences written by his contemporaries, which provide valuable insight into his activities and also reveal how he was perceived by his friends and colleagues.

The JCRS board and staff received the notice of Dr. Spivak's mission to Poland with mixed feelings. In an article titled "The Gift of the JCRS to the War Sufferers," the administration revealed it was both proud of Spivak's selection and concerned about how the Denver sanatorium would operate without him. Nevertheless, the article concluded:

> Much as the JCRS needed his valuable services at home, the trustees felt that the overwhelming catastrophe that has overtaken our brethren in war-stricken Europe required of the JCRS a sacrifice for this sacred and pressing cause. . . . Dr. Spivak's mission will be analogous to that of General Gorgas in Panama. He is to devise ways and means of suppressing disease and bringing health and strength to our stricken co-religionists. . . . His record of achievement in the campaign against the White Plague in the face of heavy odds is a good criterion of what he will accomplish in his present larger field of endeavor.[3]

The article emphasized Spivak's suitability for the task, including his medical erudition; familiarity with the language, customs, and "psychology of our Polish and Russian brethren"; and particularly his human sensitivity, warmth, and cordiality—what was labeled the "JCRS spirit." The author maintained that "Dr. Spivak has been the leading exponent of this JCRS spirit," and coupled with "his tireless energy and wonderful resourcefulness, his boundless enthusiasm and breadth of vision . . . his fellow workers were loath to have him depart, even temporarily, from their midst." As editor of *The Sanatorium*, Spivak held to a firm policy of never publishing flowery, complimentary articles about JCRS officers or trustees, but the temporary editor asserted that he had decided to violate this sacred rule "at the risk of getting fired or executed on the spot when the boss gets back." Spivak was due credit in his lifetime, the acting editor maintained, as a critical player in the JCRS's founding and development, as a man who served not only in a medical and leadership capacity but also as "[t]he office manager, general utility man, the individual to whom the applicants told their tales of woe—in short, the Pooh Bah—the 'let-George-do-it' man on whom almost everything was saddled."[4]

Spivak's departure was marked by a hasty but elaborate send-off given by "Denver Jewry." He was the guest of honor at a kosher banquet on the

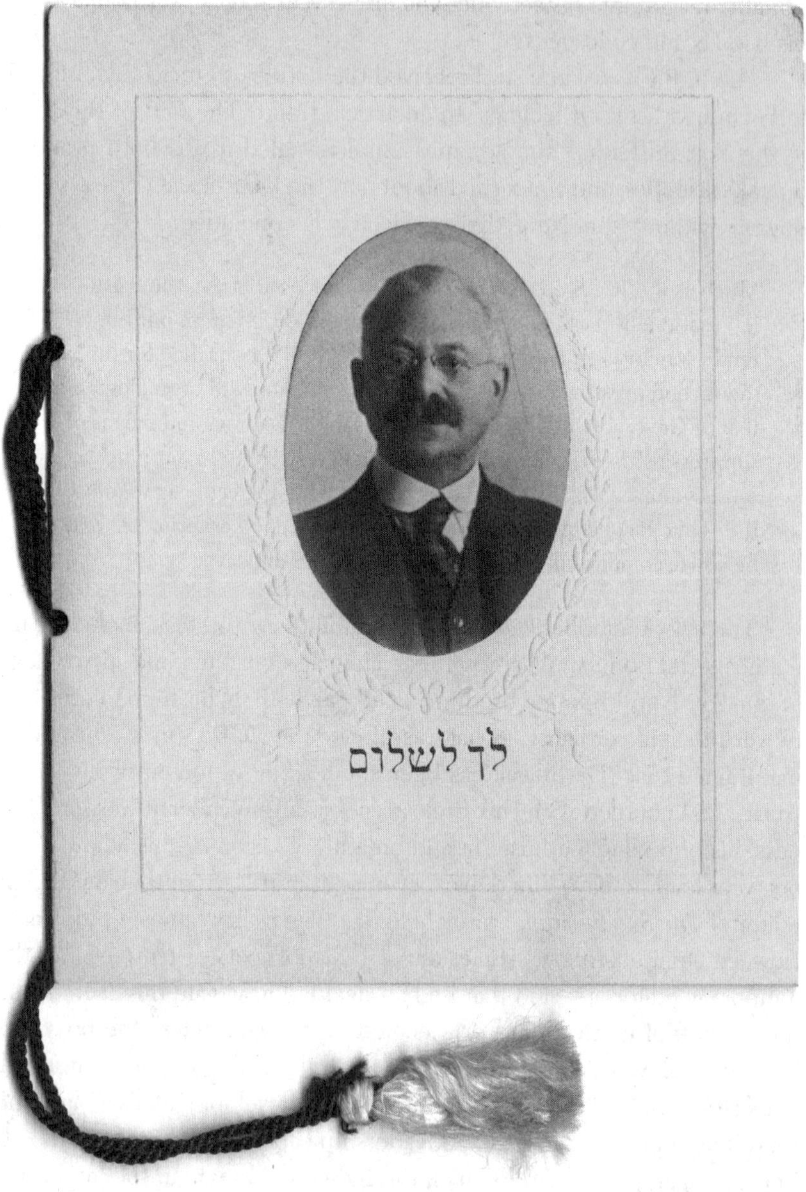

Cover of program commemorating Dr. Charles David Spivak's send-off dinner before he left for Poland, December 28, 1919. Courtesy, Beck Archives, Special Collections, Penrose Library, University of Denver.

JCRS grounds, with numerous tributes to Spivak coordinated by the toastmaster, Dr. Philip Hillkowitz. Rabbi Charles Kauvar delivered a speech, as did several local physicians, Jewish community leaders, and patients. We are fortunate that a copy of the dinner program still exists. The cover of the booklet features a formal head-and-shoulders portrait of Dr. Spivak looking uncharacteristically stern, with his mouth set in a straight line under his bushy moustache and his eyes serious behind wire-rimmed glasses. The Hebrew words "Lech L'Shalom" (go in peace) are engraved under the portrait. Each speaker and the title of his or her testimonial are listed, and the sometimes tongue-in-check headings reveal both Spivak's personality and his central role at the JCRS. Rabbi Kauvar's speech was titled "The Spirit of the J.C.R.S. and Its Oracle," and office manager Henry Schwartz called Spivak "The Idealist and Realist of the J.C.R.S." Spivak, who generally shunned the limelight, replied with a "Come Back" speech and was presented with a gold watch, engraved with the JCRS seal, in appreciation for his many years of service to the sanatorium.[5]

Following the banquet, Spivak was feted by a large crowd at Denver's Jewish Progress Club, a gathering place for Denver's Jewish upper class, where he was presented with a "handsome steamer robe" from the Central Jewish Aid Society and the Central Jewish Committee, as well as a camera from the JCRS office staff. On behalf of Denver's Jewish community, the Central Jewish Council sent an effusive letter about Spivak to the Joint Distribution Committee. "Although Denver Jewry will surely miss Dr. Spivak," it read, "we realize that this great Jew, Chaim David Spivak, who from his shoulders and upward is higher than many of the majority, does not belong to this community. . . . [W]e [therefore] say go to your noble mission."[6]

Respected social worker and educator Dr. Boris Bogen, who became the general director of the JDC's European relief society and coordinated the organization's first unit of social workers sent to Europe in 1919, referred to Spivak's role in the project in his own memoirs. Bogen recalled Spivak's initial connection with the JDC: "As a special commissioner on health work, we had with us Dr. Charles D. Spivak, founder and secretary of the great sanatorium at Denver, a devoted, dynamic, and fiery protagonist of social work for and by the masses, an ardent nationalist, a lovable personality. When the call for overseas workers had gone out, Dr. Spivak had wired for details as to what his position would be and what the conditions

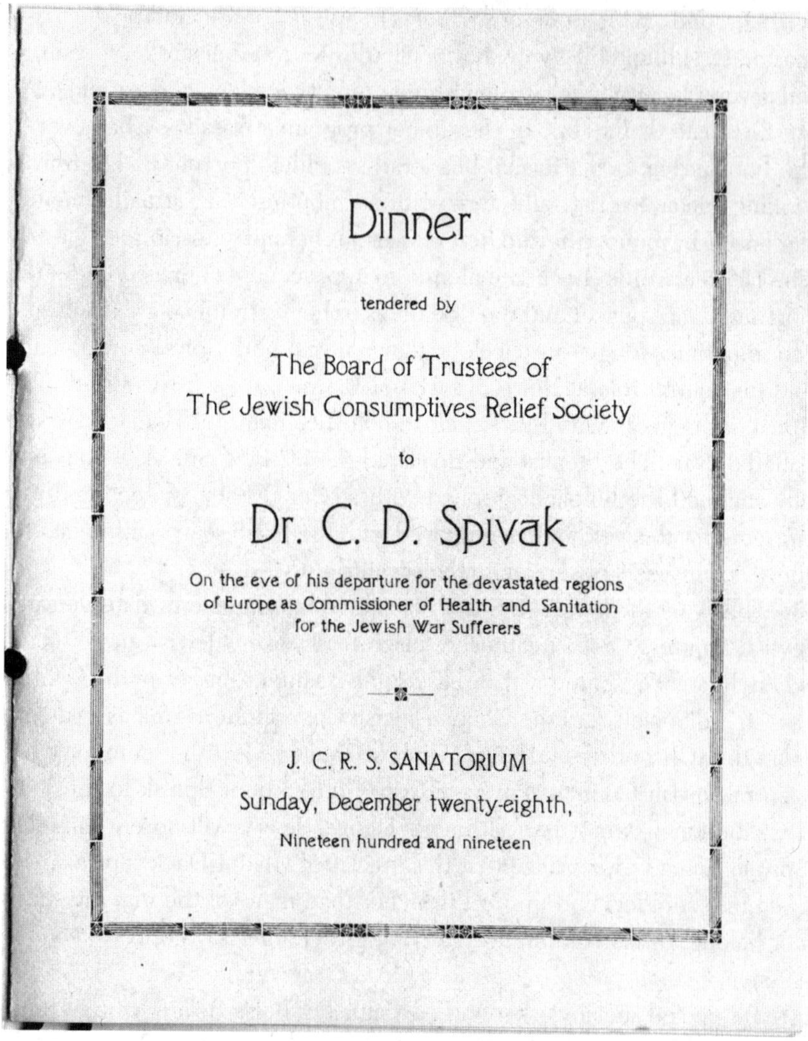

Dinner

tendered by

The Board of Trustees of
The Jewish Consumptives Relief Society

to

Dr. C. D. Spivak

On the eve of his departure for the devastated regions
of Europe as Commissioner of Health and Sanitation
for the Jewish War Sufferers

J. C. R. S. SANATORIUM
Sunday, December twenty-eighth,
Nineteen hundred and nineteen

Dinner program frontispiece, December 28, 1919. Courtesy, Beck Archives, Special Collections, Penrose Library, University of Denver.

of service would be." Bogen recounted that he replied rather harshly to Spivak's inquiry, annoyed that the question might have implied that Spivak was interested in a stipend, an honorary title, or both. Bogen informed Spivak that they were looking for workers "who desired to serve sufferers overseas without thought of honor or reward." Spivak at once offered an

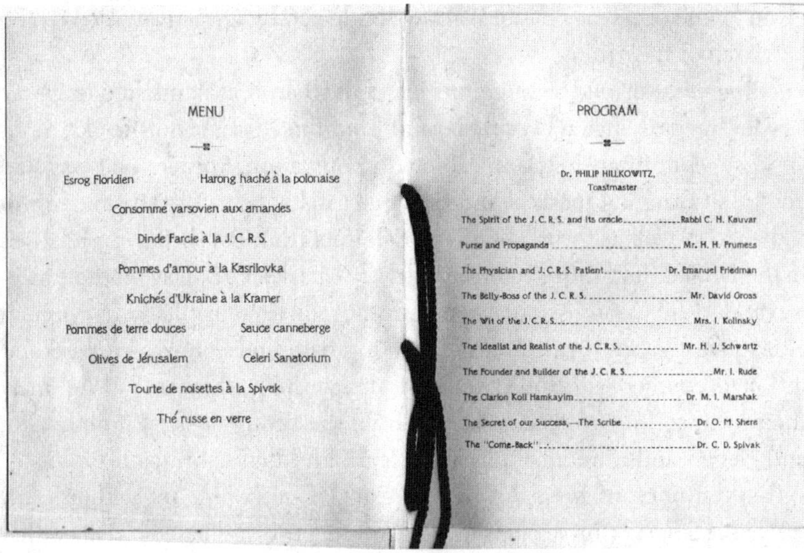

MENU

Esrog Floridien Harong haché à la polonaise

Consommé varsovien aux amandes

Dinde Farcie à la J. C. R. S.

Pommes d'amour à la Kasrilovka

Knichés d'Ukraine à la Kramer

Pommes de terre douces Sauce canneberge

Olives de Jérusalem Celeri Sanatorium

Tourte de noisettes à la Spivak

Thé russe en verre

PROGRAM

Dr. PHILIP HILLKOWITZ,
Toastmaster

The Spirit of the J. C. R. S. and its oracle .... Rabbi C. H. Kauvar

Purse and Propaganda .... Mr. H. H. Frumess

The Physician and J. C. R. S. Patient .... Dr. Emanuel Friedman

The Belly-Boss of the J. C. R. S. .... Mr. David Gross

The Wit of the J. C. R. S. .... Mrs. I. Kolinsky

The Idealist and Realist of the J. C. R. S. .... Mr. H. J. Schwartz

The Founder and Builder of the J. C. R. S. .... Mr. I. Rude

The Clarion Koll Hamkayim .... Dr. M. I. Marshak

The Secret of our Success,—The Scribe .... Dr. O. M. Shere

The "Come-Back" .... Dr. C. D. Spivak

Program for Dr. Charles David Spivak's send-off dinner. Courtesy, Beck Archives, Special Collections, Penrose Library, University of Denver.

apology for the misunderstanding, and according to Bogen, "Dr. Spivak, finely and greatly, had implored me to take him on any terms, so that he might atone, through service, for the moment that he had hesitated."[7]

Spivak's service was both exhilarating and draining. He was nearly sixty at the time, the oldest member of the staff of the medical/military operation. Further, the mission was inherently dangerous because of rampant disease, unsanitary conditions, and political unrest in Poland as a result of the war. By 1920 Spivak's reddish-blond hair was receding and turning gray, as was his trademark bristly mustache, but the twinkle remained in his blue eyes. According to a memorial article Bogen wrote after Spivak's death in 1927, Spivak's conduct during his mission was in keeping with his character, for Spivak tried to address a difficult situation with his usual efficiency, empathy, and cheerfulness. "Dr. Spivak from the very beginning and throughout the entire stay chose to serve as a private and did not want any special consideration," observed Bogen. "He strictly followed the discipline and obeyed orders without murmur. He was beloved by the boys. They looked to him for advice. . . . I shall never forget the [Passover] Seder given by the overseas boys in Warsaw conducted by Dr. Spivak. He was the patriarch of the group."[8]

Bogen described a dangerous incident when Spivak insisted on going to Kiev, recently taken over by Poland from the Russian Bolsheviks, to investigate conditions for the local Jewish population. Spivak's unit was successful in bringing medical and financial assistance to Jewish residents in the area, as well as forwarding 20,000 letters from Polish Jews to relatives in the United States. Bogen reported that "Charles D. Spivak, in the capacity of Medical Commissioner, spent most of the time in villages, towns and cities investigating institutions, collecting data and coming in close and intimate contact with the people. He knew the problems, and he knew their local setting." Spivak returned from the taxing mission in ill health, and Bogen and a military physician feared he had contracted typhus or suffered a nervous breakdown as a result of overwork. Yet within a few days Spivak's fever broke, he recovered his energy, and he complained that he had wanted to go on to the city of Jitomir from Kiev to provide further service. But the captain of the unit insisted they return to Warsaw because he felt Spivak was too worn out to continue.[9]

The conditions in Poland were appalling, and the magnitude of the public health and economic issues was overwhelming to Spivak. Yet he managed for the most part to remain cheerful; as he once wrote in an editorial in the JCRS *Sanatorium*, "the editor [Spivak] admits [to] being guilty of a streak of optimism in his makeup."[10] While in Poland, Spivak wrote a number of letters to his family in Denver, some of which were published in *The Denver Jewish News*. According to Jennie Spivak, she suggested the publication of the letters to Hattie Friedenthal, editor of the newspaper. Ill and in distress, Hattie was unable to write her usual editorials and turned to her friend Jennie for assistance. Jennie "told her not to worry. I would bring the Doctor's letters about the work of the JDC and she could use those instead of local stuff. The Denver community would be very glad to know what is going on in the world."[11] In one letter that appeared in May 1920, Spivak wrote from his hotel in Minsk, which had neither heat nor a shower or bathtub: "I am stopping at a hotel which I know will make me a fertile soil for cooties. All I hope is they be of a benign kind and not infected with typhus. . . . The people everywhere are ready and willing to help. Physicians in Minsk are very kind and organized a meeting which I addressed."[12]

Despite the trying conditions, there appear to have been enjoyable aspects to Spivak's stay in Minsk, and his reputation as a leader in the American medical and Jewish communities preceded him. Spivak recounted:

> Dr. Bogen arrived yesterday morning and I surprised him by meeting him at the depot. . . . All the prominent people of the city show me courtesies. The high officials come to invite me to all public functions. I had the [Jewish holiday of] Purim at the home of the head of the Jewish Geminde, Dr. Chargrin. . . . A Zionist meeting was held and I addressed them. . . . [S]o you see that besides my medical work, I kill time by being lionized somewhat. . . . What makes me great . . . is because I am coauthor with Yehoash of a Yiddish dictionary. The dictionary is known wherever I come.[13]

Although Spivak indulged in a bit of uncharacteristic vanity in his remarks, they were also interwoven with his usual humorous and self-deprecating style, thereby effectively taking him back down a peg.

In his formal report on the mission, Spivak concluded that the scale of need was so great it was beyond the capability of the JDC to address, but he emphasized that there was an educational component the organization could assist with. "What Poland needs most is not only a program of sanitary equipment, bathing facilities, etc.," he maintained, "but a program of Health Education." Spivak's twenty-page report reflected not only his outlook on social work but his entertaining writing style as well. Far from dry, the paper presents a lively picture of the struggles and suffering Spivak encountered in war-torn Poland. The "Confidential Report Dated Warsaw, April 13, 1920 from Dr. Spivak" began with an introduction that related that he had focused on Jews in Poland based on data he had collected in Warsaw, Wilno (Vilna), Minsk, Bobrujsk, and other sections of the country, as well as Polish-occupied Ukraine. He introduced a "personal element," as he put it, "by describing the evolution of the trend of thought which I underwent since I have been called to this work."[14]

Spivak admitted that when he first received his special commission from the JDC, he had only a faint idea of what his course of action was going to be. In the few short weeks before he received the confirmation of his position and his sailing on the S.S. *New Amsterdam* on January 10, 1920, he was focused on organizing his affairs in Denver in preparation for his absence. Only on the ship was he able to compose a plan of action.

After the three-week-trip he arrived in Warsaw on January 31, when he hoped to begin an investigation of local Jewish health care institutions with the assistance of two Warsaw Jewish physicians, a Dr. Goldflam and a Dr. Bychowski.

However, when he arrived he found that the country was devastated by a widespread typhus epidemic. As Spivak put it, it seemed "unworthy" to gather statistical information when "people were suffering and dying by the thousands." Instead, Spivak contacted members of the American Typhus Commission to offer his medical services. While waiting for the military/medical unit in Wilno, which arrived two weeks after Spivak did, the doctor filled in the time by visiting a local Jewish hospital. He "was horrified by the contrast it presented with the hospitals as they exist in the U.S." Patients were subject to unsanitary conditions reflected in the filth, odor, mold, and the lack of ventilation, proper toilet facilities, and adequate bedclothes that assaulted Spivak when he inspected the "inferno" that passed for a medical institution. To his horror, conditions at the local Jewish Home for the Aged and various orphan asylums were dire, as food was in short supply, although he was heartened by the existence of a general Wilno's Children's Hospital and clinics that ministered to the young in a much more adequate manner.[15]

While Spivak continued to wait for the military unit to join him in Wilno, he turned his attention to the study of tuberculosis in the country, an illness that had played such a central role in his life and career. After intricate calculations, he estimated that several hundred members of the city's Jewish population of 65,000 to 70,000 would die as a result of the White Plague during the year of his visit and that nearly 500 active cases were present. Typhus was even more prevalent. Spivak, realizing that he would be able to make little headway against either disease, searched for a project in which he and the JDC could have a positive impact on the state of Jewish health care in Poland. He meticulously conducted a careful and extensive survey of the entire Polish Minsk district, visiting more than 1,000 households.[16]

Spivak's conclusion was at once both startling and mundane: he attributed most disease of all kinds among Polish Jews primarily to a lack of cleanliness and what he termed "dirty habits." This was especially painful to Spivak on a personal level because he felt Jewish religious tradition and specifically the Bible emphasized cleanliness. He concluded that "it becomes a matter of great surprise, chagrin and heartache to find that the Polish Jews of the present day have fallen so low." Borrowing the term "class-consciousness" from the "Marksusts [Marxists]" as he called them, Spivak maintained that Jews were a "religious," "zdokah [charitable]," and "knowledge-conscious" people and had—prior to centuries of persecution—also been a "cleanliness-conscious" people, a character trait that had to be restored. He declared that similar sanitary issues existed worldwide wherever Jews were currently suffering from "unfavorable economic conditions."[17]

As usual, Spivak was ready with a list of recommendations to remedy the situation, but as he stated they hinged on one primary theme: "the waging of a campaign against dirt in Poland." Speaking before a group of eminent Jewish doctors in Warsaw, Spivak expounded upon his theory of cleanliness-consciousness, which resulted in the organization of the Society for Practical Hygiene. Spivak, a consummate organizer, urged that a public bathhouse under Jewish auspices be constructed, and he even managed to locate a local donor to provide the necessary funds, but at the same time he urged sanitary workers to be sensitive to the feelings and possessions of the poor Jews at whom the campaign was aimed. To this end, he proposed that Jewish health institutions be established in areas where Jews resided throughout Poland to train health agents interested in social welfare work. These quasi–"social workers" were to become public health representatives and present classes on hygiene, sanitation, and cleanliness to the masses. He maintained that the battle against typhus and tuberculosis was best left as a national project under Polish authorities, although he made general recommendations for founding several institutions geared toward guarding against infection by building up the immunity of Jewish children though milk stations and better clinics and day nurseries.[18]

In these recommendations Spivak was strongly influenced by Progressive-Era notions about the efficacy of education in treating all types of social ills. American reformers had seized upon a "gospel of cleanliness" as a central tenet in an effort to create "good citizens" and uphold "civilization" among the urban poor, many of them immigrants who dwelled in crowded tenements. Like the Polish Jews Spivak was describing, poor Americans in the late nineteenth and early twentieth centuries "faced a shortage of private bathing facilities," and public baths were seen as a means of upgrading public health.[19]

In addition to addressing public health issues in Poland, seeing the suffering of so many European children firsthand may have prompted Spivak to engage in a significant project to provide homes for many Jewish children who had lost their parents in the war. Characteristically a man of action, he searched for a practical plan. According to one source, working through the Canadian government Spivak was the agent for the relocation of approximately 250 orphaned children to that country.[20]

While Spivak was in Poland, the JCRS experienced a fire that destroyed the main building of the sanatorium. Spivak cabled as soon as he heard the news, offering his sympathy as well as a generous contribution to the rebuilding fund. When representatives of the administration expressed the sentiment that they wished he was back to lend his guiding hand, Spivak is said to have replied that the organization was bigger than any one individual and that the quick response of JCRS friends and trustees to the tragedy demonstrated that work was being carried on satisfactorily. The acting editor of *The Sanatorium* disagreed. In an article that featured a prominent photograph of Spivak in Europe posing with "A Group of Intellectuals of Kief [sic]," the editor maintained that "[w]hile in a sense he is right, men of special talent in social service work are rather rare and cannot easily be spared. . . . [W]e hope to have Dr. Spivak back at his desk in October."[21]

In the same issue, the JCRS *Sanatorium* inserted a last-minute announcement concerning Spivak's anticipated return from Europe. "As we go to press a cable from Paris announces that Dr. C.D. Spivak will sail for New York September 26th," it read. "The office force of the J.C.R.S. and the editorial staff will heave a sigh of relief on his return. It goes without saying that the patients and the Sanatorium administration will give him a hearty welcome. Lastly, our membership will be gladdened by his resumption of the correspondence and secretarial duties which will again assume the old-time pep and vigor."[22]

In the late summer/early fall 1920 issue of *The Sanatorium*, a headline declared "Dr. Spivak Home Again" and reported:

> The thousands of members, friends and co-workers of the JCRS will rejoice with the board of trustees and the office staff that the genial secretary has safely returned from his humane though perilous mission abroad and is again occupying his accustomed swivel chair in the office evolving plans and policies for the betterment of our organiza-

> tion. . . . Sobered by the sad sights witnessed among our suffering brethren abroad—scenes that transcend the description of a Dante or a Milton—he is again bending to his task of succoring the victims of the White Plague in this blessed land.[23]

In his annual president's address, Dr. Hillkowitz referred to Spivak's mission as "the Gift of the JCRS to the Jewish War Relief" and lauded him for "performing yeoman services to restoring health and life to our brethren suffering from disease and starvation. . . . The JCRS is gratified at having contributed indirectly through Dr. Spivak its quota to this great cause."[24]

Back at the JCRS Spivak resumed his duties, including his work as editor of *The Sanatorium*. In the first issue published after his return, he greeted his old friends with the customary Jewish salutation Shalom Aleichem (peace be with you). He soon turned his hand to a humorous send-up of life at the sanatorium titled "When the Editor Is Away." Although Spivak was saddened by the loss of the main building, he was elated to see that the structure of a new building had begun to take shape, as well as the erection of the two-story Rude Home a mile from the sanatorium. A number of former JCRS patients, Spivak reported, were now happily housed in a "post-graduate school for our regular health students." Spivak revealed that it was his close friend Dr. Hillkowitz who had served as the mysterious unnamed editor of *The Sanatorium* while he was in Europe. He good-naturedly chided Hillkowitz, "the unprincipled temporary editor," who had violated Spivak's firm rule never to extol the virtues of any JCRS leader in the official publication. Hillkowitz, he complained, "singled out the secretary, upon whom he heaped praise undeserved and adulation unmerited. It will take time, effort, and fumigation to cleanse the atmosphere and reintroduce the old moral standards."[25]

The same issue of *The Sanatorium* reprinted an article by Dr. Spivak titled "Health and Sanitation in the War-Stricken Countries." A popular iteration of his formal report for the JDC, the essay emphasized the centrality of proper sanitation in the health crusade and declared, "[s]trange do the words 'Health and Sanitation' sound when they are uttered in the same breath with the words 'in war-stricken countries.'" He noted the acute lack of housing in Central Europe as a result of shelling, as well as the curtailing of bathing facilities and lack of clothing. "Many persons, mostly children, go around with rags wrapped around their feet," he mournfully reported, and "the poor man has not enough bread. . . . I know people who have not had the taste of meat, eggs or butter for six months and many children have not had a drop of milk." Disease was rampant because of inadequate sanitation, housing, and nutrition.[26] Although Spivak's article was not prescriptive, it was meant to bring the plight of war victims to the attention of JCRS supporters in the hope that they would make contributions toward amelioration of the conditions.

Dr. Charles Spivak was indeed relieved to be home but grateful to have had the experience of a lifetime. His work in Europe for the JDC effectively merged several different strands of his persona and enhanced and broadened his reputation both in America and internationally. A formal head-and-shoulders photograph of Spivak in his official U.S. military uniform appeared in a number of publications around the country. The mission to East Europe on behalf of American Jewry in the region where Spivak was born demonstrated his commitment to the general Jewish community and particularly to his co-religionists who had remained behind and suffered the ravages of war. Since the project was officially under the aegis of the U.S. military, Spivak was also demonstrating a self-sacrificing, patriotic commitment to his adopted country. Because of his fluency in Yiddish, Polish, and Russian, Spivak was a valuable member of the humanitarian team, and the project offered him a chance to repay in small part the blessings America had bestowed upon him. Finally, the trip to Poland appealed to Spivak's interest in medical science and particularly public health, an area that occupied a central role in his work at the JCRS.

Spivak returned to Colorado in the fall of 1920, exhausted but exhilarated, ready to resume his multitude of duties at the JCRS as a key player in the American tuberculosis campaign. Throughout the late teens and 1920s, Spivak frequently traveled the country to attend conferences and conventions associated with a variety of organizations—Jewish, secular, and medical in nature. During this period his national reputation grew even stronger as he became associated with several key organizations within the American Jewish community. Dr. Spivak served as a delegate to the American Jewish Congress (AJC), organized in 1918 with the goal of creating a national Jewish democratic organization composed of Jewish leaders from throughout the United States. The AJC was primarily devoted to securing equal rights for all Americans. Spivak also became a member of the Executive Committee of the American Jewish Committee, formed in 1905 to protect the rights of American Jews, and he served in this capacity

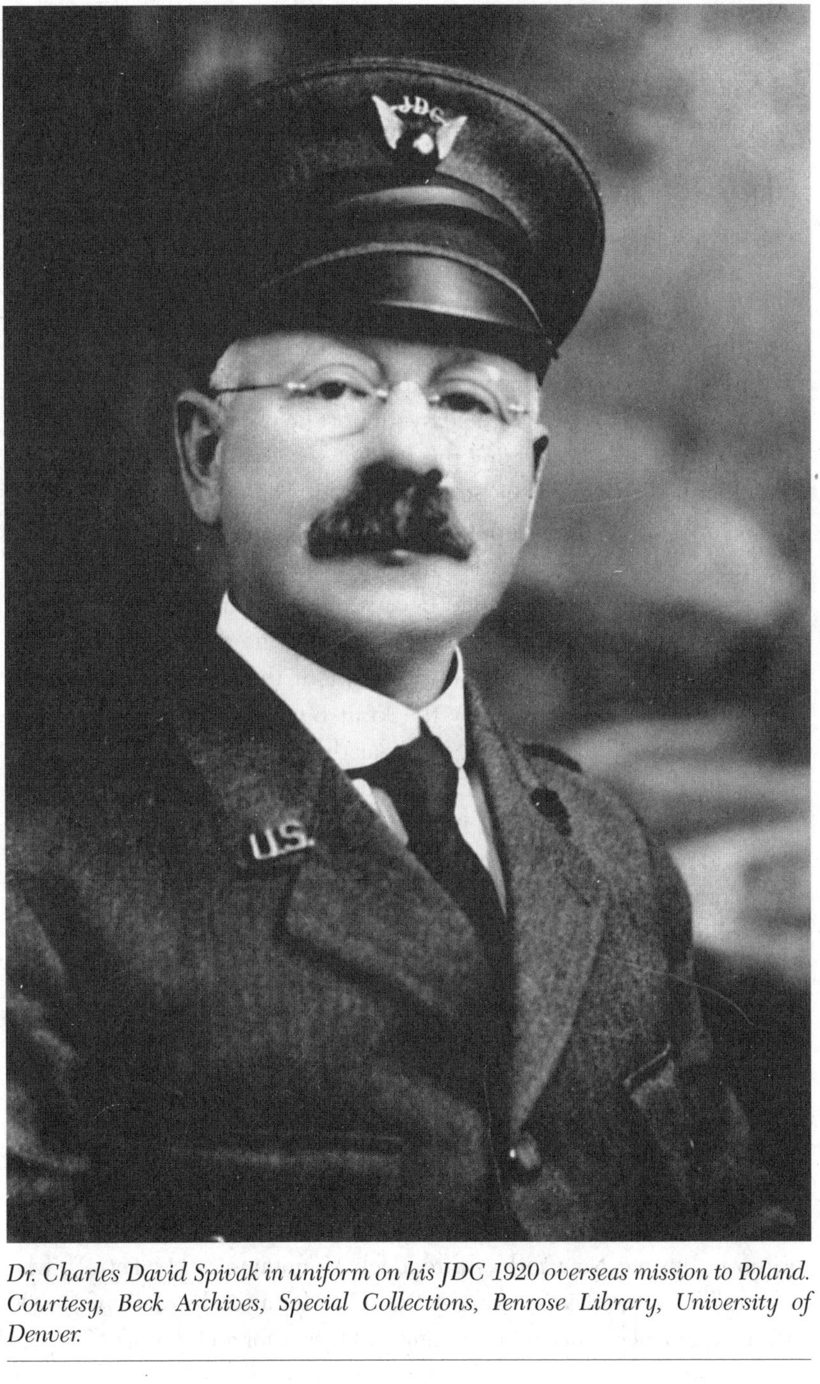

Dr. Charles David Spivak in uniform on his JDC 1920 overseas mission to Poland. Courtesy, Beck Archives, Special Collections, Penrose Library, University of Denver.

from 1914 until his death. Spivak crisscrossed the United States on many occasions in his capacity as a community leader and on behalf of the JCRS. Between May 27 and June 9, 1916, for example, Spivak took advantage of a trip to Pittsburgh for the JCRS annual meeting to stop in Kansas City and St. Louis on the way to make "illustrated lecture" appearances on behalf of the JCRS. Following the Pittsburgh event he traveled to New York City to meet with JCRS representatives.[27]

Spivak also attended all the annual conventions of the JCRS, which were held in a different U.S. city each year, and he took a key role in planning the events. Spivak's special report on the plenary meetings for the upcoming 1922 Boston convention reflects his high energy level, his ability to juggle many tasks, and the easy rapport he was able to maintain with all types of people. Addressing the JCRS Executive Board in Denver, he noted that he had arrived in Boston on the afternoon of March 23, 1921, and was met at the train depot by several JCRS supporters. In his signature humorous style, he reported that the evening's meeting of the Board of Directors was poorly attended because "it was raining pitchforks" and it coincided with the Jewish holiday of Purim. "The reformed and the orthodox National Directors were busy," he wrote, the former occupied with attending a dance sponsored by the local B'nai B'rith organization and the latter gathered in synagogues to hear the traditional recitation of the biblical Book of Esther to honor the holiday. The meeting was rescheduled for the following Sunday, when it was well attended. Spivak used his diplomatic and organizational talents to form a volunteer committee. Ever the realist, he noted that "the work of the [volunteer] Committee, no matter how well selected, must be carried on by a paid official," and he hired a young local law student to fill the position.[28]

Following days filled with meetings and negotiations in Boston, Spivak took the train to New York City, where at the JCRS Medical Advisory Board's request he continued to search for a qualified scientist to conduct tuberculosis research at the Denver sanatorium. To that end, he had interviewed several candidates in Boston and then at the Bedford Hills tuberculosis sanatorium near New York City. Spivak finally located the most promising candidate after a long journey to Trudeau's famous Saranac Lake sanatorium in upstate New York's Adirondack Mountains. A Mr. Petroff, who indicated his interest in working at the JCRS for a yearly salary of $5,000 and "maintenance," was to be brought to Denver for an interview.[29]

While in New York, Spivak also attended dozens of meetings with representatives from the New York office of the JCRS in regard to their general work as well as one of his pet projects, the organization of "health circles," where "meetings should be held at regular intervals at which the subject of health and the prevention of the disease [tuberculosis] should be presented by competent lecturers. The Secretary [Spivak] laid the foundation for such a movement in the near future."[30] Spivak's interest in the health circles reflected the larger issues of tuberculosis and public health in which he was involved. The American tuberculosis movement was one of the first successful examples of a national public health campaign, and Charles Spivak was one of the leading proponents of the associations created in its wake.

Spivak's close friend Isaac Rivkind, of the Jewish Theological Seminary in New York City, recalled that wherever the doctor traveled he brought along his ongoing magnum opus—a bibliography of Jewish medical works, which he was still compiling shortly before he died. "He was really always on the go," Rivkind wrote, "with one foot on the train, and the other in the 'tent of the law,' in the library, at the writing table."[31] Spivak's longtime friend Dr. A. Levinson of Chicago reinforced this observation, maintaining that "[i]n his travels from place to place he always carried with him a copy of the Bible in Hebrew. In every city to which he went he sought out the library, where he could be seen poring over books that would add to his knowledge of Jewish lore."[32] When Dr. Spivak was in the throes of a writing project, time had no meaning for him. According to Rivkind, it was not uncommon for Spivak to compose an article by working the entire night, "sitting at his desk until dawn, and on the next day [he] resumed his work on behalf of the Sanatorium."[33]

In his later years, one of Spivak's most charming writing projects was a series of popular articles on health and hygiene written for the Jewish daily *The Forward* (*Forverts*), which was edited by his good friend Abraham Cahan. As a highly successful "ethnic broker," Spivak often used his literary talents to help Americanize his fellow East European Jewish immigrants, but he did so in a style laced with gentle humor so they were made to feel that his prescriptive instruction was given in an affectionate manner and that he and his readers were equals. As we learned in Chapter 2, Spivak and Cahan shared a common immigrant background and commenced their lifelong friendship on the journey to America.

In the United States, Cahan had honed his journalistic skills as a reporter for New York newspapers before striking out on his own in 1897 to found *The Forward*, which ultimately served as an information source, teacher, and counselor to hundreds of thousands of Jewish immigrants. In short, the paper's underlying goal was to help readers find their way in a new land with a new language and often different customs. While the political bent of *The Forward* and its socialist editor Cahan was decidedly to the left, the publication encouraged immigrants to become full American citizens and to take advantage of new civic responsibilities and opportunities. Its popular "Bintel Brief" (Bundle of Letters) section was a prototype "Dear Abby" column that dispensed practical advice to its readers. At its peak in the 1920s, the Yiddish-language daily paper had more than a quarter of a million readers around the country and was one of the first U.S. newspapers to go national.[34]

Cahan, who became famous as a novelist and whose best-selling book *The Rise of David Levinsky* became an emblematic recounting of the clash between the Old World and the New in the American immigrant experience, stayed in touch with Spivak over the years. In 1921 Cahan saluted "Dr. Chaim Spivak from Denver, Colorado" in an article in *The Forward* on the occasion of the latter's sixtieth birthday. The piece featured a photograph of a beaming Dr. Charles Spivak in uniform on his trip as special medical commissioner to Poland, discussed earlier in the chapter. "Everyone knows him," maintained Cahan. "And were he not so modest, much more would be known about him. To know him is to love him. There is no lovelier nor more beautiful person, not in America, not in the Old Country."[35]

From April through June 1922, an article written in Yiddish by Spivak appeared each week in *The Forward*. Each essay focused on advice for good health and longevity and specifically tied good habits to prescriptions from the Torah, the Talmud, and the book of Proverbs. As Spivak became reconnected to the traditional Jewish roots he had experienced as a child in Russia, he increasingly became convinced that the Jewish Bible provided the source for all wisdom, including in the areas of medicine and health. *The Forward* consciously tried to coach readers about health so they would become familiar with American middle-class urban values regarding hygiene. To this end, Spivak's articles were thoughtfully labeled with provocative and humorous titles to attract immigrant Yiddish-speaking readers and draw them in so they could be inculcated with what we would today consider "proper" middle-class American values. Some of the more interesting titles were "Dr. Spivak Proves That All the Commandments of the Torah Are Designed to Prolong Life," "Washing Hands Is Not Only a Religious Observance," and "Don't Crawl into a Clean Bed with Dirty Feet."[36] As a physician, Spivak firmly believed that ignorance about cleanliness and hygiene resulted in the unnecessary spread of many diseases, including tuberculosis.

From his first days in Denver, Spivak had always maintained a hectic schedule, and family obligations often weighed heavily upon him as far back as the 1880s, when he was a struggling medical student in Philadelphia. However, despite a lifetime of challenges, undoubtedly one of the most painful episodes in Charles Spivak's life occurred in 1922, when his wife, Jennie Charsky Spivak, began displaying symptoms of mental illness and instability, manifesting in erratic behavior.

The first hint of overt difficulty appeared in a letter dated March 20, 1922, from the Spivaks' old friend in Chicago, Dr. M. Sahud, who had boarded in the Spivak home as a young medical student. Jennie had arrived to visit the Sahud family. According to the story she told Sahud, she was there for a "rest and change after a slight attack of 'flu'" on her way to tour New York, Palestine, and Europe. In the letter Sahud described his concern over Jennie's apparent transformation from a "kind, practical" individualist and was clearly alarmed that "her nervous condition of late years" had made her appear "fanatical" and unstable. "And with all her altruistic tendencies," Sahud wrote, "she is still under the struggle of her old individualism ('I'm perfectly free'—'no boss over me,'—'the children don't need me anymore,' and 'I can go wherever I please' etc.)." Sahud went on to say that only two days into the visit Jennie had decided to go ahead to visit her daughter Ruth, who was living in New York City, and that he hoped "a loving conspiracy with Ruth" would convince Jennie to return to Denver for help.[37]

Within a few days Jennie had traveled to New York to join Ruth and May Schwatt, Jennie's sister and the wife of Dr. Herman Schwatt, who had served as the medical director of the JCRS from 1910 to 1915 (a position he would resume for a few years after Spivak's death). May was Jennie's youngest sister and had shared her interest in acting. Under the name May Arno, May had traveled as an actress with a theater company in the early years of the twentieth century, and while residing in Denver she had run a dramatic arts school for children. While her husband served as the JCRS's medical director, May turned her hand to writing on behalf of the organization. In 1911, under the appellation May Arno Schwatt, she penned a dramatic story titled "The Violinist's Last Hour," the tragic tale of a twenty-two-year-old consumptive violinist who died soon after entering the JCRS.[38]

As soon as Jennie arrived in New York City, May wrote her brother-in-law Charles Spivak a reassuring letter:

> She is calmer and more quiet and composed than she has been for years. . . . The reason she left Chicago so soon is because Ruth and I thought that as long as she is not at home and in that strained condition in which I found her in Denver, she would be better off here with us, and it proves to be so. As for Ruth, she is old enough and sensible enough with a little help from me to be able to carry on her own work undisturbed and help her mother. There is absolutely no necessity for you to worry about her acts here. So far she spends all her spare time with us, and it seems to have a quieting and good effect on her. . . . Thanks so much for the Schalech Mones [traditional gifts of food sent on the Jewish holiday of Purim]. It was very thoughtful and kind of you to remember us at this time. With love, May.[39]

But the calm time did not last, and in September Dr. Schwatt sent Charles Spivak a frantic telegram advising him that "Jennie apparently very sick previous trouble." He went on to say that Jennie was living in a rooming house and refused to stay with the Schwatts. "We are helpless and dreadfully worried. Come at once," pleaded Schwatt. This time the illness seems to have had a physical component, as Spivak received another note at the same time, presumably from two New York physicians: "Mrs. Spivak has [had] one of her heart attacks. Besides she is extremely nervous . . . her condition does not permit letting her travel by herself."[40]

Spivak rushed to New York, where Jennie had been admitted in the interim to Bellevue Hospital. The forty-eight-year-old "housewife," as she was termed, was listed as suffering from "mental trouble." According to her record, she was released into the custody of her husband to return to Colorado, where she entered Woodcroft Hospital in Pueblo.[41] In a series of letters, Dr, C. W. Thompson, the medical superintendent at Woodcroft, reported on Jennie's condition, which varied weekly between cheerful and restless but overall seemed to show "some improvement." The monthly cost for care at the hospital was $150, but that charge had been reduced to $100 as a courtesy to Spivak because he was a physician. It was still a considerable sum for a man of modest means.[42] During October May Schwatt wrote several letters to Spivak expressing interest in Jennie's progress and her hope that "Jennie will get over this."[43]

The following month Jennie's condition continued to fluctuate, but by mid-November Dr. Thompson was able to report that she was "getting along quite comfortably and she is showing improvement . . . and I think she will recover from this attack. However, it will probably be necessary for her to remain under treatment for some time."[44] Although no exact treatment plan or diagnosis was forthcoming in any of the medical reports, at the time Jennie's condition might have been termed "hysteria," today perhaps seen as bouts of serious but intermittent depression experienced over several years.

Jennie recovered her health to the degree that she once again became active in family and community affairs, and her grandchildren's memories provide additional insight into her personality as well as that of Spivak. Her granddaughter Adele Strauss Karsh and grandson Eugene Spivak remember her as a vibrant, energetic, and opinionated woman who was a great fundraiser and dedicated volunteer on behalf of the JCRS. Jennie remained vigorous and alert until her death in 1965 at age ninety-six. Adele also recalled that family lore suggested Jennie's illness was merely the result of a "difficult menopause," but most family members agree that she had some sort of breakdown in the 1920s, albeit short-lived. Although Adele and Eugene were only eight years old when their grandfather died, Adele recalled "Papa" Spivak as an extremely warm, mild-mannered individual who never raised his voice. Even when the dramatic Jennie would "rant, rave, and holler," Adele maintained that Dr. Spivak would calmly answer, "Yes, *lieblich*; yes, dear."[45]

Although the Spivak's youngest granddaughter, Charlesa Wolfe Feinstein (named after her grandfather), was born after Dr. Spivak's death, she has clear memories of her grandmother as a highly intelligent, independent, and strong-minded woman. When Charlesa's father, Dr. Joseph Wolfe, served as a medical officer during World War II, she, her mother, Ruth Spivak Wolfe, and brother David moved from Texas to live with her grandmother in Denver at the South Franklin Street home for several years. She remembers Jennie Spivak as still a spry, fun-loving woman who appreciated opera, continued to read widely, listen avidly to the radio, and remained abreast of current events even in her later years.[46]

A few years after the difficult period in Jennie's life, Spivak received a letter from his brother-in-law Dr. Schwatt informing him that he was not "*broigez* [angry]" at Spivak because the latter was unable to visit him when last in New York City: "You are such a bird of passage when you come east that you must be forgiven." Although Schwatt went on to say that their paths had become so divergent that they no longer had much in common, he concluded by saying, "I continue to wish you good health and a little happiness but I know you won't get it—it's too late,"[47] perhaps a veiled reference to Jennie's illness.

Still, despite personal challenges and worries over Jennie, Charles Spivak remained active not only in the JCRS but in the national social work arena and the Zionist movement, as well as in his literary and scientific efforts. Perhaps the stress impelled Spivak to become even more involved in professional matters to distract him from his home life. In a memorial written after Spivak's death, Dr. Sahud alluded to the unsettled period in Spivak's life and how he met the challenge. "I do not know of any one who could do such serious work, necessitating deep mental concentration, under the most adverse and unfavorable circumstances, as did Dr. Spivak," Sahud observed. "He could be under great mental anguish and suffering, and yet his work was not left undone. A few years ago when a member of his family was acutely ill, and Dr. Spivak was on that account, under a tremendous mental strain, he worked on a very important scientific problem."[48]

While Spivak sometimes disagreed with family members over their actions, politics, or ideology, his loyalty appears to have been unshakeable. This was evidenced in his student days when he cared for his elderly mother, and it resurfaced graphically in the light of Jennie's illness. Although Jennie's breakdown may have been exacerbated by hormonal changes and perhaps by her husband's long hours away from home on behalf of the JCRS and myriad other projects, from a young age she appears to have exhibited a volatile, sometimes tempestuous personality.

As Jennie improved, the 1920s became an especially prolific period for Spivak. His goal of addressing social issues on a national scale led him to become very prominent in the National Conference of Jewish Social

Service (NCJSS), an organization that focused on Jewish philanthropic agencies and the emerging field of social work. In June 1924 he traveled to Toronto to attend the NCJSS conference and spoke about Jews living in Soviet Russia at the time. Spivak was active in organizing the annual meeting of the National Conference of Jewish Social Service, held in Denver in June 1925. At the meeting Dr. Spivak was elected a national vice president of the organization, and he was listed on the stationery as one of three national vice presidents until his death in 1927. The Executive Committee included well-known leaders within the American Jewish community such as jurist Julian Mack, philanthropist Cyrus Sulzberger, and banker Felix Warburg—all from New York.[49]

Although Spivak favored centralized organizations as effective in many cases, one notable exception was his antipathy for federated Jewish charities. Dr. Spivak's views about the concept of federated charities evolved over the years. In 1921 he published a lengthy essay on "the Federated Jewish Charities Movement in the United States" in the JCRS *Sanatorium*. Spivak's careful outline notes for the article are preserved in his distinctive hand and reflect his organized thinking and writing process and the careful manner in which he approached a writing project.[50] In the published article, Spivak criticized the federation movement for separating the giver from the receiver and for being undemocratic by disenfranchising the poor from participation in the support of charitable institutions. Instead, Spivak called for a community movement modeled on the traditional centralized Jewish *kehillah* that had existed in Europe, where he maintained that historically, communal funds had been distributed equitably to provide the needy with food, clothing, medical assistance, burial of the dead, education, and shelter, among other functions. According to Spivak, the emphasis on community over federation did away with bureaucracy. Spivak concluded that the "[f]ederation is only a stepping stone to the *kehillah* movement" and that several truly national organizations such as the JCRS and National Jewish Hospital deserved support from the wider Jewish community because they in fact were "owned" and populated by Jews from all over the United States.[51]

Of course, Spivak had a vested interest in the subject, which hardly made him an impartial observer. He felt that "national" organizations like the JCRS should have the ability to conduct private fundraising in cities throughout the country and not be subject to restrictions imposed on sanatorium fundraisers by local federation rules. As head of the JCRS fundraising team, Spivak was confident that he could raise more than the modest allotments local Jewish federations were willing to dole out to the Denver sanatorium.

A prolific letter writer, Spivak had first taken the opportunity to discuss his vision with his old friend and leading Jewish social worker Dr. Boris Bogen of New York. Spivak sent an advance copy of his article to Bogen with the request, "I know that you are a very busy man and it is an imposition to make you read in addition to the reading you are doing from early morning until late at night, and yet I ask you to do me a favor and peruse the enclosed advance copy of *The Sanatorium*."[52] Without waiting for a reply, Spivak dispatched a copy of his proposal.

Bogen not only read the essay but sent a lengthy critique to Spivak highlighting his own views: "As usual, I am very much impressed with your presentation but inasmuch as you are inviting my comments, will you permit me to say a few words which will give you my opinion on the subject." Bogen maintained that he did not think the federation was a forerunner of the *kehillah* movement, as they were very different in "principle and construction." The federation was not a democratic entity, as it was managed and directed by large subscribers, whereas the *kehillah* looked to the entire population for the selection of its leaders. One of the strengths of the federation, in Bogen's opinion, was that its collection program saved time and reduced duplication. Despite Bogen's differences of opinion with Spivak, however, he supported the doctor's strong feeling that "national" organizations such as the JCRS should not affiliate with federations and should instead be permitted to "organize in the field" and "raise your own funds."[53] Spivak was understandably so pleased with Bogen's view on this matter that he republished the letter in full in the next issue of *The Sanatorium*.[54]

Although Spivak liked to debate philosophical issues nationally, it was at home at the JCRS that he put his progressive social views into practice. As an innovative "social worker," Spivak tried to secure funds to give patients a new start after they left the JCRS. He also advocated training patients in such trades as printing and bookbinding, which would not tax their strength but would provide them with the means to make a living once discharged. Spivak was proud of the 1924 launch of the Rude Home, supported by prominent Denver Jewish immigrant philanthropist Isadore

Rude, nicknamed "the Little Tailor." Spivak described the project as a boarding home for former patients that would not only provide housing at a very modest cost but would also be supervised by physicians. He noted sadly that many former patients were subject to relapses because the stress associated with finding accommodations and competing for work placed them in a precarious position. By providing proper medical supervision and easing their "economic" burden, the Rude Home would help prevent breakdowns and launch former patients on the path to maintaining their health.[55]

Spivak was equally proud of the Max Neusteter Rehabilitation Building, completed in 1926. The new facility, which housed a bookbindery and printing shop, had long been located in the basement of the main building. As H. H. Frumess, chair of the rehab committee, reported, the program had three main purposes: occupational therapy, industrial rehabilitation, and employment for former patients.[56]

Charles Spivak's ties to Palestine and his interest in Zionism were germinated while he was still a student in Russia and came to fruition in Denver. As early as March 1912, prominent Denver attorney Philip Hornbein had invited Spivak to serve as a member of the Denver general committee for the United Palestine Appeal, which had a national goal of raising $7.5 million.[57] By the next month, Dr. Spivak had personally contributed $100 toward the Rocky Mountain region quota of $10,000—a significant sum at the time, considering his modest income.[58] A 1918 letter from the New York–based Palestine Bureau to Spivak attested to the doctor's continued financial support of "New Zion" through purchase of a land certificate.[59] The certificate indicated that the land was purchased for $250, and in 1924 it was determined that Spivak was entitled to "five dumas . . . equal to about five city lots of 20 × 100."[60]

With his close friend Rabbi Kauvar of the BMH Synagogue, Spivak endeavored to arouse Zionist sentiment in Denver. Following World War I, Jews across the country gathered to urge the recognition of a Jewish state at the Paris Peace Conference. As an officer of the Denver Zionist group, Spivak used his considerable persuasive powers to author an ad published prominently in November 1918 in *The Denver Jewish News*: "Are You with the Allies and the USA in the Peace Conference? Their Program Demands Autonomy for All Peoples Including a Home Land for the Jewish People." The ad was signed by the Zionist Organization of America Colorado

Registration Committee, C. D. Spivak, Treasurer.[61] Spivak's profound attachment to Zionism continued as the years passed. In February 1925 the Denver Hadassah group held a "propaganda" meeting in an effort to promote the women's organization. "On that occasion we shall have the leading Jews of this city express their views in regard to Zionism. Would you be willing to be our main speaker for the affirmative side?" Spivak was asked by the event's chairwoman.[62]

Spivak served on the national Board of Directors of the Zionist Organization of America. In the summer of 1925 he was invited by Felix Warburg to become a member of the American Advisory Committee of the Hebrew University in Palestine, a significant recognition of his stature, as Warburg was one of the most widely respected figures in the American and Jewish communities. The Hebrew University had been dedicated in 1918 by Dr. Chaim Weizmann and counted among its founders Weizmann, Albert Einstein, and acclaimed New York rabbi and Jewish community leader Judah Magnes.[63] Spivak's boyhood friend Victor Yarros maintained that "he [Spivak] was in his last phase a fervent Zionist, and talked to me with enthusiasm of the Palestinian colonies and the spiritual as well as economic significance of the movement for a Jewish homeland and a State." Although Yarros was skeptical about the entire subject, Dr. Spivak continued to try to persuade his friend of the soundness of the idea and frequently sent Yarros articles to help convince him to support the cause. Spivak's style was to present a well-organized and thoughtful argument but to let individuals come to their own conclusions.[64]

As time passed, Dr. Spivak continued to be a popular speaker nationally as well as in Denver, and his early foray into amateur acting in Philadelphia stood him in good stead. Spivak's lively and entertaining lectures were always well attended, and he spoke before Jewish, gentile, and medical audiences alike. Dr. Spivak is said to have presented a yearly lecture at Denver's BMH Synagogue, where his close friend Rabbi Charles Kauvar was the spiritual leader, and in 1925 Spivak presented a lecture on "Diet and Nutrition" to the Young Women's Christian Association of Denver.[65] He remained on the cutting edge of medical thought as well, and toward the end of his life he was advocating medical specializations in both neonatology and gerontology, new fields at the time. In the same article, Dr. Spivak documented about 1,800 practicing physician in Colorado engaged in a variety of specialties.[66]

Dr. Spivak's early socialist ties have been discussed at length and were closely related to the support the JCRS received from national unions and workingmen's organizations. In Denver his solidarity with workers was evidenced in his close association with the small local branch of the Arbeiter Ring (Workmen's Circle). The national Arbeiter Ring was founded in 1892 as a fraternal organization for radical socialist secular Jews. Dr. Spivak was a frequent speaker at local meetings, and in 1919 a lecture series featuring Spivak and several other physicians associated with the JCRS was noted in *The Denver Jewish News*.[67] As a testimonial to Spivak's contributions to the organization, after his death an educational building was erected in Denver by the Arbeiter Ring, dedicated as the Spivak Institute in his memory.[68]

Denver was the site of few garment factories in the first decades of the twentieth century, so it is not surprising that the city did not feature a significant Jewish labor movement, prominent in other large urban centers such as New York City and Chicago. It is noteworthy that a small trade union—the Journeymen Tailors' Local—was created at the JCRS in 1916. This occurrence was proudly reported in *The Denver Jewish News*, edited by Dr. Spivak at the time.[69] Tailoring and the needle trades had been the major occupations of many JCRS patients. Between 1904 and 1923, 21 percent of the sanatorium population listed tailoring or a related job as their source of income, followed distantly by clerks, who comprised only 14 percent of patients.[70]

Connected to his affinity for the Jewish labor movement, Spivak was also involved in creating Denver's short-lived Yiddish School, organized largely on secular lines. However, once again reflecting Spivak's evolving religious views, he pushed for the introduction of biblical stories and familiarity with Jewish holidays to foster religious culture among the children as well. From 1917 until about 1923, following the formal organization of Denver's Workmen's Circle branch, a successor school came into existence.[71] In the year before his death, Spivak helped found the Non-Partisan Jewish Workers' Children's School. Classes, which included instruction in Yiddish, were held at the Labor Lyceum located at Julian and Conejos streets in Denver's west side immigrant community.[72]

Just months before his death, Dr. Spivak—labeled a dreamer by an early friend and colleague—was still hatching plans for numerous projects, including several articles and a new sanatorium on the East Coast. In

July 1927 he felt well enough to drive his wife and daughter to Colorado Springs for an outing to celebrate the Fourth of July,[73] a favorite holiday of Spivak's, who appreciated the opportunities America had afforded a poor Russian immigrant. His work in the American West had brought Spivak acceptance and acclaim from his peers, and his name had become well-known nationally. Moreover, in the fluid and open society of early Denver, he was treated as an equal by his non-Jewish colleagues.

The last of Dr. Charles Spivak's many publications was an article titled "Longevity according to Hebrew Lore and Tradition," which appeared in the April 1927 issue of *Medical Life*. Spivak's typescript copy still exists in his personal files. As was his norm, to the end Spivak linked his interest in medical history to Jewish subjects. In the essay Spivak traced several Jewish cultural influences that he maintained contributed to a longer life among the Jewish population. One theme, he noted, was that "[t]he Jews have a peculiar attachment for medicine as a science. They have an extraordinary respect for physicians, and according to testimony of physicians, both Jewish and Non-Jewish, the Jews as a group avail themselves of the services of physicians more frequently and more readily than any other group in the world." Moreover, Spivak reported that beginning in the Middle Ages, there was a higher proportion of doctors among Jews than among any other group, reflected in quantifiable statistics. Spivak attributed these proclivities to the high rate of literacy among male Jews at least and their multilingual exposure—which often included Hebrew, Yiddish, Aramaic, and the language of their host country—as well as biblical prescriptions that stressed proper living.[74]

From his youth until the end of his life, Spivak was a "literary man" who was constantly refining his views through reading and writing. No matter how busy his day, how complicated his personal or professional life, books, periodicals, and his own written work remained an integral part of his life. When one reads his articles and essays today, his style remains fresh and appealing. We are indeed fortunate that his "writer's itch" was never cured. Spivak's outlook on life may have evolved over time, but at heart philosophically he remained an "optimistic" Jewish reformer, albeit one who came to accept gradual, measured progress as his creed.

8

Conclusion: The Spivak Legacy

Dr. Charles David Spivak approached his final illness in the same manner in which he had faced the many vicissitudes of life: with determination to rise above his challenges and move forward, buttressed by the company of family and friends. Indeed, adaptability and versatility, coupled with a quest for knowledge and empathy for others, were the fundamental elements of his personality. Even in his last days—ill with terminal liver cancer—Spivak's sense of humor, philosophical stoicism, and calm acceptance surfaced in a letter in which he informed a friend of his disease:

> Well, you may just as well learn it from me that unless a miracle is performed the days of the writer of these lines are numbered. I was operated for gallstones July 21. Was delivered of the grand total of 613 stones of all colors and dimensions [613 is the traditional number of *mitzvot*, or commandments, in the Torah]. . . . On the same date there came two physicians (the Assistant Surgeon and Dr. Hillkowitz), both solemn

> and apologetic, and after preliminary remarks in which my philosophic attitude toward life was extolled, they informed me that at the time of the operation it was found that I suffer from primary carcinoma of the liver. . . . So, that is that! . . . [I] [w]alk around. Read a good deal. Enjoy the visits of friends.[1]

Jennie Spivak traveled to New York City to be with her husband as he pursued radiation therapy for his cancer. Sadly, the treatment was unsuccessful. The couple returned to Denver, and Charles Spivak passed away on October 16, 1927. In his honor, the Workmen's Circle later erected the Spivak Institute building as an educational facility on Denver's west side, where part of Spivak's personal library was housed. Bearing a plaque that bore the inscription "The Charles D. Spivak Educational Institute," the small edifice served as the site for numerous literary lectures and musical performances.

Spivak's religious beliefs had always been complex, a fact brought to light again at the time of his death. His highly unusual instructions for his burial were highlighted in local newspapers, and *The Rocky Mountain News* quoted his will directly: "It is my will and direction that my funeral shall be conducted with Orthodox Jewish rites and ceremonies. It is my will that no addresses or eulogies should be delivered at my funeral." The newspaper reported that the will had been witnessed by two of Denver's most prominent Jewish attorneys, Theodore Epstein and Philip Hornbein.[2] Epstein became a member of the Board of Trustees of the Beth HaMedrosh Hagodol (BMH) Synagogue and had been appointed by the Colorado State Supreme Court to its grievance committee. Hornbein, an ardent Zionist and supporter of the Jewish Consumptives' Relief Society (JCRS), was considered one of Colorado's outstanding trial lawyers and had led the fight against the Ku Klux Klan in the state in the 1920s. Despite Spivak's emphasis on simplicity at his funeral, over 6,000 people attended, and nearly 2,000 were present at a memorial meeting held at the Broadway Theatre thirty days after Spivak's death to mark the end of the traditional thirty-day Jewish mourning period of *shiloshim*. At the Broadway Theatre assembly, Hornbein eulogized Spivak as "the personification of democracy" and "a man who gave his heart and his soul to save human life."[3]

The Rocky Mountain News noted that Spivak's further request in his will to have his body dissected contradicted Jewish law, but "although he pitted science against religion," according to the newspaper, it was "in the cause of aiding humanity."[4] In November 1927 the newspaper ran an article titled "Autopsy at Colorado Medical School Witnessed by 125 Doctors and Students," which recorded the dissection procedure that had been carried out according to Spivak's wishes. Spivak's longtime friend, pathologist and JCRS president Dr. Philip Hillkowitz, defended Spivak's request, claiming that his will reflected both Spivak's love for Judaism and his firm belief that "autopsy was a sign of respect for the dead in the interest of learning more about illness to help the living."[5] Even in death, Spivak was still struggling to negotiate his sometimes competing religious and scientific sensibilities.

Shortly after Spivak died, noted Denver gentile physician Dr. Henry Sewall penned an editorial titled "Concerning Spivak" in the December 1927 issue of *Colorado Medicine* that revealed the high esteem in which Spivak was held by his non-Jewish colleagues. Sewall, who had migrated to Colorado because of tuberculosis, was a cardiologist and professor of medicine at the University of Colorado.[6] In the article, Sewall described an experiment Spivak had conducted on musical sound shortly before his demise, which was published in the journal *Science* on October 21, 1927, just days after Spivak died. Sewall concluded with a fitting epitaph: "For originality in thought, for initiative in execution, for unselfish devotion to the general welfare, for the naïve enthusiasm when new truths lurked, we shall not soon again see the likes of Charles D. Spivak."[7]

In a lifetime filled with many accomplishments, the Jewish Consumptives' Relief Society ultimately served as a testimony to Charles Spivak's greatest achievement as an acknowledged and critical weapon in the war to conquer tuberculosis that reflected his agenda of social and medical reform. Although Spivak's articulated skeleton was to be shipped to Palestine to serve as a teaching aid at the University of Jerusalem, he had also requested that his viscera be buried in the Workmen's Circle section of the Golden Hill Orthodox Jewish cemetery, near his deceased JCRS patients. Visitors to Denver can still visit the gravesite today. In the ethical will in which Charles David Spivak left careful instructions for his burial, he is said to have remarked in Yiddish, "*Ikh vel zey bashaynen, zey veln mir bashaynen*" (I will beautify them, and they will beautify me), referring to the patients next to whom he had requested to be buried.[8] Even at the end, Charles Spivak managed to merge his love for humanity, medicine, Jewish tradition, and his socialist roots.

A few days after Spivak's death, on October 20, 1927, Denver's *Intermountain Jewish News* printed an effusive eulogy and detailed description of his funeral. "For three decades, Doctor Spivak was a beacon and stimulus to American Jewry, and the pulse of the Sanatorium of the Jewish Consumptives' Relief Society, which he founded in Denver in 1904. The welfare of humanity was the aim of his efforts. To the patients of the hospital which he fathered, he devoted his ideal during his lifetime," the paper observed.[9] The Philadelphia *Jewish Exponent* declared that "Dr. Spivak's love for humanity did not extend to his co-religionists alone. His heart went out to every suffering human regardless of creed, sect and nationality."[10]

While Spivak's funeral, conducted at the BMH Synagogue by his old friend Rabbi Charles Kauvar, was simple according to Spivak's express instructions, throngs of admirers—Jews and non-Jews alike—paid their respects, making it one of the largest in Denver's history. Following the service Spivak's coffin was driven to the JCRS, where the pallbearers, who included Dr. Philip Hillkowitz and Dr. Emanuel Friedman (who had volunteered his services to the JCRS and become one of Denver's most beloved pediatricians), carried it to the Solarium building. There, the JCRS patients, many of whom had developed close relationships with Dr. Spivak, participated in the emotional mourning rites. Finally, the remains were driven past "every building of the sanatorium, the buildings that owed every brick to Dr. Spivak's life efforts," before being interred at Golden Hill Cemetery, about three miles west of the JCRS off West Colfax Avenue. The Jewish press throughout the United States "was unanimous in paying tribute to Dr. Charles D. Spivak."[11]

He was perhaps most intensely mourned at the JCRS. "Dr. Spivak's rare qualities, his indomitable energy and enthusiasm, his ceaseless love and concern for his suffering fellowmen has [sic] left an ineradicable impression upon the JCRS. The history and growth of the JCRS and its Sanatorium is [sic] inseparably bound up with the self sacrificing work of Dr. Spivak."[12] That is how Dr. Charles Spivak was described in a booklet *Thirty Years of Saving Lives,* published by the JCRS in 1934. Years after his death, Spivak was still acknowledged as the guiding genius and heart and soul of the institution's development.

Soon after notice was given of Spivak's passing, memorial services were held in cities and towns throughout the country. Hundreds of donations poured in for the Spivak Memorial Foundation, to benefit the JCRS, from admirers from all over the United States—including a contribution from his old friend Abraham Cahan, the famous editor of *The Forward*.[13] Spivak's files also contain numerous messages of condolence to both his biological family and his JCRS "family." According to the terms of Spivak's will, dated September 3, 1927, the sum of around $30,000 was left to his widow, Jennie, and smaller modest sums to his three children—David, Deena, and Ruth.[14]

Spivak was a human being like all others and thus not without blemishes and flaws, such as a tendency to rush headlong into new schemes, but while eulogies are notoriously praiseworthy and uncritical, in Spivak's case the accolades appear sincere and well deserved. Historians are trained to read between the lines to search for hidden agendas, but careful scrutiny has revealed few, if any, subtexts among those who wrote about Spivak after his death or even during his lifetime. The president of the National Jewish Federation for Social Service, for example, wired his sentiments: "We are sorrowfully moved at the passing of our beloved friend Dr. Spivak. May the monument which he erected in his lifetime serve as an eternal urge to all whom he inspired to work in this mission of administering to suffering humanity."[15] The president of the gentile Denver Colonnade Club honed in on Spivak's oft-noted characteristics: "Leaders are rare, and great humanitarians are even rarer. . . . Dr. Spivak, lost to us, is not only the loss of a great leader and a great humanitarian who had no equal in this city, but also the loss of a great friend."[16] Jennie Spivak received a resolution from the National Tuberculosis Association a few months after her husband's passing that attested: "In the death of Dr. C.D. Spivak the tuberculosis movement has lost a pioneer worker . . . and the Association hereby records its appreciation of the labors of Dr. Spivak."[17]

Perhaps one of the most touching and all-encompassing memorials was offered by Denver's B'nai B'rith Lodge, which had initially denied Spivak membership many years before. Prominent Denver Jewish leaders and attorneys Simon Heller, Simon Quiat, and Charles Rosenbaum recalled "the sweet, lovable traits that had endeared him to all of us. . . . He was an educator, a physician, an author, a communal worker, an indefatigable worker in all worthy causes—giving of himself and of his means. . . . He preached and was a living example of the saying 'Kol Yisroel Chaverim,' that all Jews are brothers, and all people constitute one brotherhood."[18]

While Spivak's concern for humanity as a whole found its greatest focus in aiding his Jewish co-religionists, he believed all people, regardless of race or creed, were to be treated as equals. In this, he was far ahead of his time. A very telling illustration appears in the minutes of a JCRS board meeting in July 1923, at which a "lively" discussion was held regarding the sale of the Rude Home, managed by the JCRS and located in nearby Edgewater, Colorado. A proposal was on the agenda concerning the possibility of selling the building to "colored people," a move opposed by a number of Edgewater residents. Several board members expressed the view that the JCRS should honor the residents' wishes and that not doing so might ignite discord and a "racial war" in a peaceful community. A minority group of three board members, led by Dr. Spivak, argued for the sale to members of the African American community, maintaining that not doing so "would indicate intolerance and therefore would be immoral. The Society cannot be a party to any group of people who are ignorant, bigoted and prejudiced against their fellow men who happen to have their skins colored dark. Jews, who are themselves persecuted and discriminated against, should be the last to register opposition to any group of people for no other reason than that of color." Although the minority view was voted down, Spivak's progressive views on race were clearly visible.[19]

On the rare occasions when Spivak's views did not prevail at the JCRS, he took it in stride and searched for fresh opportunities. In letters written throughout his life, Spivak was almost always positive, descriptive, and entertaining, and he revealed his underlying engaging personality. One of his regular correspondents, Samuel Micon, a JCRS supporter from Chicago, provided telling insight into Spivak's outlook on life. Micon first met Spivak in 1912, visited with him frequently at public events over the years, and corresponded with him until the latter's death in 1927. "The character of a man is best revealed by his private correspondence," Micon maintained. "In Dr. Spivak's private letters he reveals only a desire to maintain human lives." Micon was particularly struck by the fact that although men in public life frequently ran up against critics, he never encountered any detractors in Spivak's case. Micon attributed this in part to the fact that he had personally never heard Spivak criticize any individual, especially anyone associated on any level with the JCRS.[20]

In all the public memorials extended to Spivak after his death, only one was critical. In November 1927 *The Intermountain Jewish News* ran an opinion piece, with a clear disclaimer that the author's views in no way reflected the views of the paper. Spivak was never named in the essay, but the identity of the subject was clear. While the author conceded that Spivak had done much for medicine and humanity, he criticized Spivak for compromising his early radical roots: [Spivak], he complained, had "tried to live his life to please the majority" and joined all "respectable movements," such as "charitable institutions, Zionist movements, all movements which did not interfere with the present order of society."[21]

The disgruntled radical critic had perhaps failed to appreciate the transformation that occurred after Spivak's encounter with American society and western life. Although Spivak's idealism and commitment to a reform agenda were never far from the surface, he increasingly emphasized the *possible* over what *might* be. As we saw in Chapter 2, while still in Philadelphia he had counseled the young Russian writer Leon Kobrin to abandon his radical leanings for a more moderate socialism, one that emphasized what could be done to better the lives of people in the here and now over a utopian future. However far from perfect, America had offered Spivak freedom of thought and opportunities on a personal level that were only dreamed of in his revolutionary days in Russia. He became an appreciative American citizen who flourished in the generally benign democratic environment.

Still, Charles Spivak was an individual who by no means assimilated in a pejorative sense but who rather negotiated a complex identity that was at once Russian, American, and Jewish. Unlike many other first-generation immigrants who had almost entirely rejected their Jewish roots for secularism, Spivak retained his allegiance to both Judaism and his fellow Jews. Moreover, he tied his medical persona closely to both his Jewish and American facets. His life was a stark contrast, for example, to that of one of his most famous Jewish immigrant contemporaries Dr. Joseph Goldberger, born in the Austrian-Hungarian Empire in 1874. A prominent public health official, Goldberger earned national fame for his successful crusade to cure and prevent pellagra. Goldberger had followed a very different path from Spivak—marrying out of the faith, making science his primary religion, and, for the most part, distancing himself from the Jewish community.[22]

Spivak's personal odyssey from Russian radical to respected American physician followed a rather uncommon trajectory and provides historians

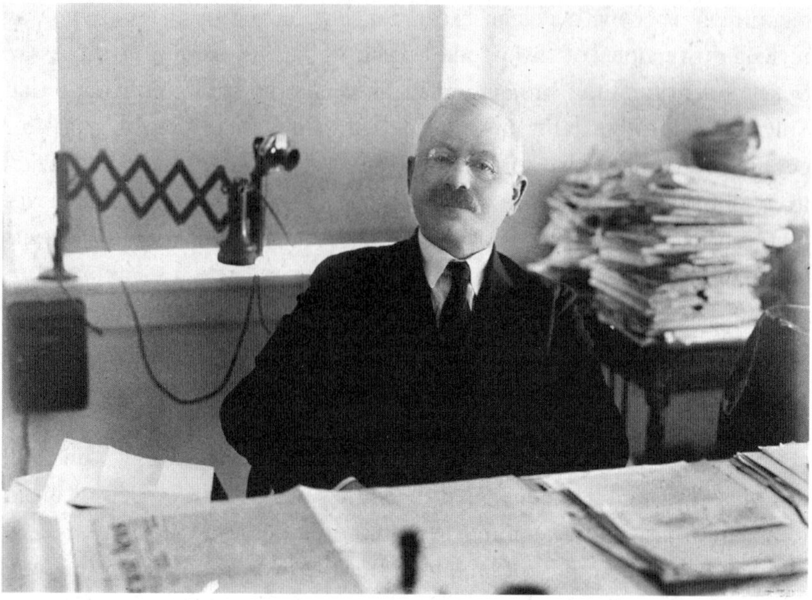

Dr. Charles David Spivak seated at his desk at the JCRS in the 1920s. Courtesy, Beck Archives, Special Collections, Penrose Library, University of Denver.

with an alternate model with which to study immigrant acculturation. It is a model that demonstrates a remarkable degree of reciprocity in which immigrants are not only influenced by the mores of the host culture but affect that culture as well. Spivak's cultural, political, and religious values resulted in a heightened sense of community responsibility at the JCRS, which addressed health issues in an inclusive manner as he merged his commitments to medicine, radical social change, and Judaism. In other words, his intellectual worldview influenced the "politics" of health care in the very fundamental way in which he practiced medicine.

Yes, Spivak had moved into the mainstream of American life. While on one level he had joined the Jewish and general establishments, he retained his cheerful skepticism as well as his close ties with the working class, which in turn continued to shape his outlook. Although he was a man of great tolerance, with, as we have seen, friends from every walk of life and ideological persuasion, at the same time he was an independent thinker who held firm convictions. As his close friend Isaac Rivkind remarked, "It would be a mistake, however, to think that Spivak was a person without a backbone. . . . It was quite the contrary. He was throughout his life a man of strong principles, adhering to them staunchly, but he was among the few blessed people, who could lift themselves above the artificial divisions of life."[23]

It is revealing that some of those who disagreed with Spivak on many subjects still forged a close relationship with him. Rabbi William Friedman, an early founder of National Jewish Hospital (NJH), had been a vocal critic of the JCRS—particularly the policy inspired by Dr. Spivak in which tuberculosis patients in all stages of the disease were admitted, even those who had virtually no hope of recovery. Many acrimonious exchanges between the two men had taken place in public venues in the early years. As time passed, however, Friedman became the doctor's close friend and admirer. After Dr. Spivak's death Friedman was quoted as saying, "His loss as it affects me is heavier than I can say."[24]

Perhaps Charles Spivak's most outstanding trait was his ability to communicate with people from all walks of life, whether through the written word, conversation, or more formal lectures and speeches. A colleague of Spivak's recalled that "Dr. Spivak was one of those rare persons who inspired confidence and friendship from the onset. His beaming smile, his warm handshake, were enough to make one feel like greeting him with '*Shalom Aleichem* [peace to you], Chaim!' Where in the world have you been all these years? Think what I missed in not knowing you before!"[25]

The story of Dr. Charles Spivak and the JCRS also offers an often overlooked perspective on western history: the American West played a central role in the American tuberculosis movement. Of those who journeyed west, many came to seek their fortunes, but a significant number—perhaps as many as a third of the migrants to the region—came to recover their health. By the end of the nineteenth century, an ever-growing number of tuberculosis victims were arriving in Colorado and other western states in search of a more favorable climate that afforded plentiful fresh air and sunshine, and many were finding a new permanent place to live as well as searching for a cure for their disease. As Rabbi William Friedman put it "The fame of Colorado's capitol [sic], nestling in a valley flooded with sunshine, protected from the extreme heat and cold, attracted not only the ambitious searcher for wealth, but the enfeebled seeker of health. . . . No wonder Colorado was a land of promise towards which tens of thousands turned their faces."[26]

As we have seen, the small Jewish community in Denver at the time reacted to this onslaught of "lungers" by founding two national sanatoriums. With the establishment of the two hospitals, the Denver Jewish community took a unique turn that profoundly influenced its demographic development. If the overall Jewish population in the West stagnated or even declined between 1900 and 1940, the special situation produced by the attraction of two Jewish tuberculosis hospitals led to a significant increase in Denver's Jewish population. Certainly, the growth of Denver's Jewish community after 1900 was stimulated by an influx of predominantly East European Jews who joined other religious and ethnic groups to "chase the cure" in Colorado's benevolent environment.[27] Many of the Jewish patients who recovered their health in either the NJH or the JCRS, together with family or friends, made Colorado their new home.

The introduction of the sanatorium on the American landscape in the nineteenth century represented the institutionalized application of science and medicine to what had been an informal rest home approach. At the peak of the tuberculosis epidemic in the early 1900s, over 200 sanatoriums of various sizes and degrees of medical expertise existed in Colorado. The sanatorium phenomenon also reflected the Progressive Era's optimistic hope that science and public education could be powerful weapons in the war on the disease to "improve the social conditions that bred the disease and control the behavior of those with the disease."[28]

From its inception in 1903, these were underlying principles incorporated at the JCRS as it grew from a local grassroots movement initiated by a group of Jewish working-class consumptives, supported by Dr. Charles Spivak and a few other local Jewish physicians, to a prominent battlefield in the national public health campaign dedicated to the eradication of tuberculosis. While the JCRS followed the national norm in many ways, it also followed a unique path that could be directly traced to Spivak's influence. "He [Spivak] was a pioneer in a new and enlightened method of healing the sick and poor," one observer wrote.[29] In other words, Spivak effectively channeled his early radical convictions into more empathetic and humane treatment of patients in general and especially toward unconventional and pathbreaking treatment for tuberculosis victims with severe cases of the disease, who had generally been marginalized by the medical mainstream. In this area in particular, Spivak was able to synthesize his

Jewish and scientific personae to forge an innovative approach that formed the heart of his life's work.

Moreover, as historian Alan Kraut has maintained, at the turn of the twentieth century "the health care field became a cultural battle among old and new Americans, and at times, even among the newcomers themselves."[30] With his medical degree in hand, Dr. Charles Spivak entered the skirmish on the side of the underdog, the ill and impoverished, most especially among his East European immigrant co-religionists. He was still fighting the battle when he died, but the odds had significantly shifted to the side of those once considered greenhorns, and the torch of leadership had been passed largely to the East European immigrants and their children.

In a speech given before a large audience of Jewish tuberculosis workers in Washington, D.C., in the spring of 1924, Dr. Spivak focused on the work the Jewish community had performed within the American tuberculosis movement. "The anti-tuberculosis treatment in the United States is only three decades old," he informed the audience. "Twenty-five years ago, almost at the very birth of the anti-tuberculosis movement, the Jews built the first sanatorium in Denver [NJH]. The Jews were the vanguard of this movement. . . . The future historian of tuberculosis will devote a chapter to the contribution of the Jews." He especially emphasized the critical role the JCRS had played in expanding humane treatment to those in all stages of the disease: "The JCRS halted this current of thought [that only early cases should be treated] by asserting that it makes no difference whether advanced cases will or will not recover, we will admit them anyhow, for it is surely the advanced case that needs more care than the early case."[31]

Spivak's strong sense of ethnic consciousness, community responsibility, and medical expertise shaped the direction of the JCRS sanatorium for nearly a quarter of a century. Under Spivak's leadership the JCRS's continuing commitment to a homelike setting and free medical services distinguished it from the typical Progressive-Era hospital. Under his aegis many JCRS patients were able to continue their traditional religious observances as they negotiated the path from immigrant to American. As Kraut has pointed out, "Cultural sensitivity is a critical adjunct to charitable assistance,"[32] and health care was a "crucial terrain" in the integration struggle immigrants experienced.[33]

These were axioms that Charles Spivak understood as paramount, and his philosophy continued to inform operations at the JCRS even after his death. In his medical outlook, he was far ahead of his time. By the time Spivak died in 1927, the self-contained JCRS "town" included a hospital, research laboratories, a cooperative store, a post office (officially named Spivak, Colorado, in 1928 in his honor), a dairy and chicken farm, a book bindery and printing shop, a library, and perhaps most notably a small but beautifully constructed synagogue—all built for the benefit of the patients.[34] What is perhaps more remarkable is that the concern for the patient as an individual lingered at the institution even as the physical campus continued to expand.

The JCRS patient population had increased by leaps and bounds over the years. In 1904 only 30 patients were treated at the sanatorium. By 1908 the number admitted rose to 242, and in 1926—the year before Dr. Spivak died—508 people entered the JCRS.[35] Ultimately, 10,000 patients passed through the JCRS. Dr. Edward Trudeau's Saranac Lake Sanitarium (the first and arguably the most famous of its kind in America) treated 12,500 patients between its opening in 1885, nearly two decades prior to the JCRS, and its closing in 1954.[36] Like Saranac Lake, the JCRS ceased to exist as a tuberculosis sanatorium in 1954 and evolved into Denver's AMC Cancer Research Center. Today the former JCRS campus, which has been placed on the National Register of Historic Places, is the home of the Rocky Mountain College of Art and Design and still features an old restored patient "tent." Dr. Spivak, the father of David Spivak, an accomplished artist, would no doubt be pleased to know that hundreds of art students weekly crisscross the campus with which he was so closely associated. Plans are also under way to restore the JCRS Isaac Solomon Synagogue.

A key question emerges as to whether the sanatorium movement, in which Charles Spivak was a key player, was successful. The answer is somewhat elusive in that the death rate from tuberculosis had already started to decline by the mid-nineteenth century, perhaps reflecting on one level the natural wax and wane of plagues and the better standard of living, particularly in America. As historian Nancy Tomes has pointed out, Progressive-Era reformers recognized a fundamental point that holds true today as well: "[I]nadequate nutrition, housing, and health care weaken natural resistance against disease."[37] Moreover, in retrospect, prevention rather than treatment appears to have been the most successful weapon in the tuberculosis crusade, although the sanatorium certainly served as a quarantine environment that restricted spread of the disease.

Even more noteworthy, between 1904—the year the JCRS sanatorium opened—and 1919, the national mortality rate for tuberculosis declined by an impressive 33 percent.[38] For many victims of the disease, the typical sanatorium combination of rest, diet, and open-air therapy, supplemented with surgical procedures, helped arrest if not entirely cure their illness. Still, not until the mid-1940s, when effective drug therapy—beginning with the antibiotic streptomycin and the drug PAS (para-amino salicylic acid) and culminating with the introduction of isoniazid in 1951—appeared, was tuberculosis considered "under control." The use of an arsenal of drug therapies that included the triple "cocktail" revolutionized tuberculosis treatment and in most cases made the need for the traditional sanatorium unnecessary. By the early 1950s most sanatoriums across the country had either closed or transformed themselves.

Dr. Charles Spivak, with his ebullient energy, had been an ideal candidate to run the JCRS, as he excelled at balancing numerous tasks simultaneously. Spivak's boyhood friend Victor Yarros recalled a visit at the latter's office in Chicago in May 1927, just months before the Spivak died, at which Spivak shared with Yarros his plans for initiating another tuberculosis sanatorium on the East Coast. Yarros reported that Spivak had been working hard and "loved his jobs—of which, as always he had several."[39] Similarly, Dr. Spivak's protégé Dr. M. Sahud, who had boarded with the Spivak family while he was a medical student in Denver, observed, "Dr. Spivak, as a worker, was indefatigable. I do not know of any man, except possibly [Thomas] Edison, who could work so much and in so many different directions."[40]

Indeed, as a man of many talents, Spivak had been involved in numerous projects while serving in the position of JCRS secretary, yet he still had a hand in virtually every aspect of the institution from the day he came onboard in 1903. In fact, the first meeting of the Board of Trustees was held on January 13, 1904, in Spivak's own medical office.[41] No detail, no matter how insignificant, seems to have escaped his attention. Each patient was greeted by a letter from Dr. Spivak "inviting" him or her to the sanatorium. In the early years, he wrote daily letters of instruction to the sanatorium superintendent from his home and office at 1421 Court Place as he juggled his responsibilities at the JCRS (unpaid for years) with his private practice. In August 1909, for example, he instructed the superintendent to replace the current *mashgiach* (kosher supervisor) with a qualified patient: "He is hereby appointed as Mashgiach, at the same salary as his predecessor."[42] Spivak's involvement in the minutiae at the JCRS did not change over time. The minutes of the Agricultural Committee meeting held in April 1925 record that on that date Spivak led a discussion on the desirability of painting the chicken coops.[43]

As executive secretary, Dr. Spivak had assumed the major responsibility for JCRS fundraising, not only personally supervising field secretaries who collected funds but also imposing his social vision on the institution. Largely as a result of Spivak's outlook, influenced heavily by his socialist ideals, the JCRS came to resemble the modern Progressive-Era hospital. Yet, in its sources of financial backing it differed radically. Most hospitals before the turn of the twentieth century depended largely on various combinations of philanthropic contributions and interest dividends, but as early as 1905 paying patients increasingly became the major source of hospital funding around the country.[44] In Denver almost all sanatoriums charged for medical care, including Swedish National Sanatorium and Lutheran Sanatorium, although some beds were set aside for charity patients who were treated free of charge. In Denver only the JCRS and the NJH treated all patients at no cost to them.[45] More than a decade after the JCRS was founded, Thomas Galbreath remarked on the expense for tuberculosis treatment in Denver, observing that the cost of care in even an inadequate boardinghouse or sanatorium ran from ten to twenty-five dollars per week.[46]

By all indications, Dr. Spivak looked upon medicine as a calling rather than a profession. This underlying philosophy informed his relationships with patients, colleagues, and friends. From his earliest days in Philadelphia, he waived fees for countless patients, and making money was a low priority. Even during the last years of his life he was still cheerfully providing advice and aid. Following a visit to a Denver dentist, Spivak received a letter from the man in which Spivak's payment check for services rendered was returned. "Now—honest, I cannot accept it ," wrote Dr. Jay Sophro, "for the reason that you have done in the past so many favors for me and my family that the little bit I have done for you last time you were at my office does not permit my consciousness [sic] to accept it."[47] In an earlier letter, Sophro revealed that Spivak had provided "generous help" to the family when Saphro's son Lincoln was dying from an undisclosed illness.[48]

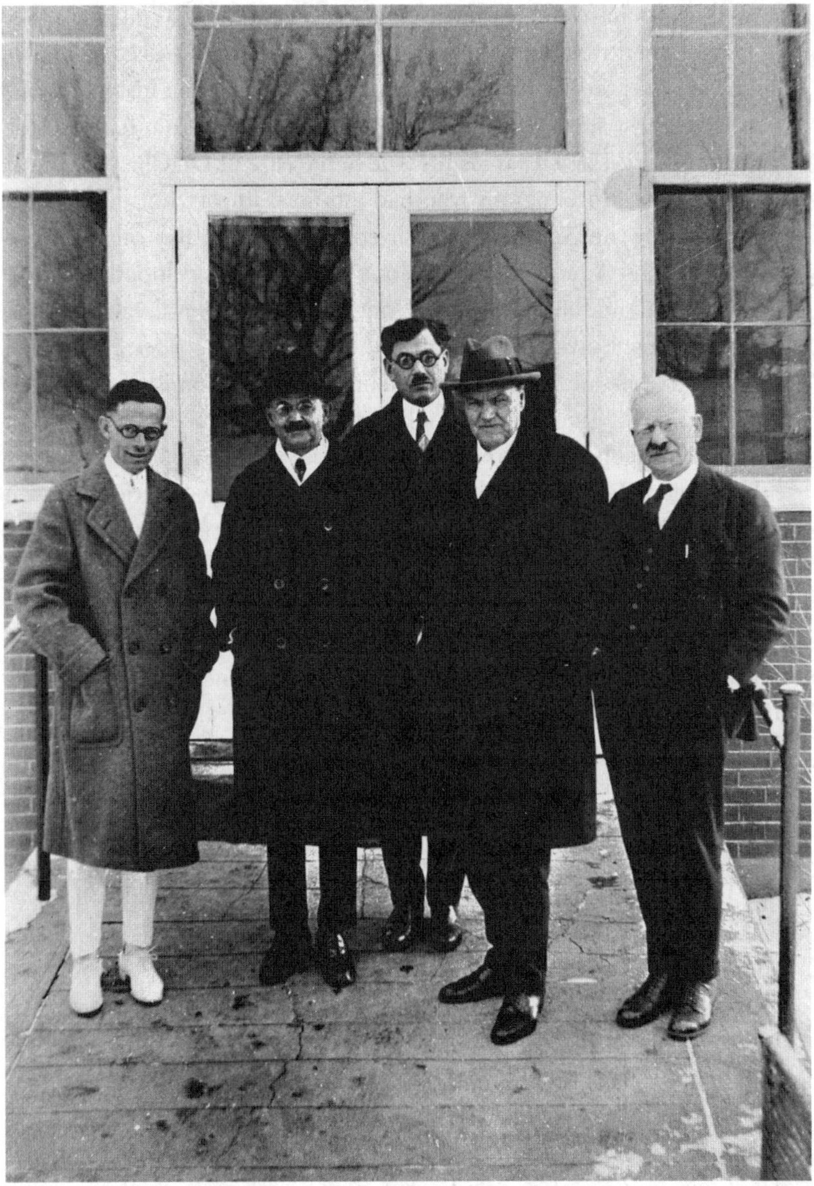

The American lawyer Clarence Darrow of Scopes trial fame visited the JCRS in 1926. Pictured (left to right) are Dr. Isidor Bronfin, JCRS medical superintendent; Denver juvenile court judge Ben Lindsey, Dr. Leo Tepley, Clarence Darrow, and Dr. Charles Spivak. Courtesy, Beck Archives, Special Collections, Penrose Library, University of Denver

While Jews have always been a minority among U.S. citizens, they have played a central role in the sphere of immigration. As historian Paula Hyman has observed, "Jews were not marginal to American history; as one of America's most successful immigrant groups, they were integral to the making of America."[49] This is visibly true in the case of Dr. Charles Spivak, a Jewish American immigrant who had a crucial impact not only on the development of the American Jewish community but also on the manner in which the American tuberculosis movement developed and how patients—immigrant and non-immigrant, Jewish and gentile alike—were treated. After Dr. Spivak's death, an editorial in Denver's *Rocky Mountain News* titled "A Life and Bequest" proclaimed: "The humanist [Spivak] was an American in the finest sense; but he was something more—he had centuries of tradition behind him, guiding his pen."[50]

The saga of Dr. Charles Spivak and his role in the American war on tuberculosis takes on special relevance today in light of the resurgence of the disease. For weeks, the story of a young lawyer from Georgia, who had contracted a drug-resistant type of tuberculosis in 2007 and then flown on several international flights, dominated newspaper headlines and television and radio news. Ironically, more than a century after Denver's National Jewish Hospital had opened to treat and eradicate tuberculosis and over fifty years after "effective" antibiotics to fight the disease appeared on the horizon, the hospital was back in the limelight treating the infamous patient. Learning about Spivak's work in the tuberculosis movement connects us to the ideas of the past and graphically illustrates that public health and medical issues often seem to resonate and echo over time. Then, as now, prevention rather than treatment appears to be the key to eradicating infectious diseases.

Once again, questions are being raised about the nature of the illness, its transmission, and effective treatment. And once again, health concerns are being tied to themes of immigration, migration, and concerns over national security and civil liberties. Spivak's life story took shape against the backdrop of many contexts and sheds light on a number of crucial currents in late-nineteenth- and early-twentieth-century America—most notably urbanization, industrialization, massive immigration, and the transformation of American medicine. He is best remembered for his dedication to treating patients, no matter their class, ethnicity, or religious affiliation. Like his more famous contemporary Jewish immigrant Albert Einstein,

Spivak was a nonconformist and an independent thinker but also a man who appreciated order and the benefits of religion.[51] Throughout Spivak's extraordinary life, he remained a man of boundless energy, an independent and creative spirit who thrived on new ideas and projects. Above all, Dr. Charles David Spivak was dedicated to the noble undertaking of saving lives, and his life has much to teach us about honoring individuals and their cultural traditions while providing state-of-the-art but sensitive medical care.

Notes

CHAPTER 1: INTRODUCTION

1. After he received his medical degree, Spivak was usually referred to as Dr. Charles David Spivak or Dr. C. D. Spivak. In the interest of efficiency, he will generally be called Dr. Charles Spivak in this book.

2. Interview with Deena Spivak Strauss, in Jeanne Abrams, *A Pioneering Legacy: An Early History of the Jews of Colorado* (Denver: Rocky Mountain Jewish Historical Society, 1988), on deposit in the Beck Archives, Special Collections, Penrose Library, University of Denver (hereafter Beck Archives).

3. *The Sanatorium* 22 (October–December 1927): 2, Box 170, Beck Archives.

4. For comparative information on Jews, Italians, and a variety of immigrant groups, see Roger Daniels, *Coming to America: A History of Immigration and Ethnicity in American Life* (New York: Harper Perennial, 1990).

5. Alan M. Kraut, *Silent Travelers: Germs, Genes, and the "Immigrant Menace"* (New York: Basic Books, 1994), 155–157. Immigrant Jewish physician Dr. Maurice Fishberg was moved to write an article to refute the stereotype titled "The Relative

Infrequency of Tuberculosis among Jews," *American Medicine* 2 (1901): 695–699. In a later article on the same subject, "Tuberculosis among the Jews," *Transactions of the Sixth International Congress on Tuberculosis* 3 (New York, 1908): 415–428, Fishberg reported that at the beginning of the twentieth century the percentage of Jews with pulmonary tuberculosis was only 13.1 percent, compared with 24.6 percent for Protestants and 49.6 percent for Catholics.

6. Nancy Tomes, *The Gospel of Germs: Men, Women, and the Microbe in American Life* (Cambridge, Mass.: Harvard University Press, 1998), 11.

7. S. Adolphus Knopf, *Tuberculosis as a Disease of the Masses and How to Combat It* (New York: M. Firestack, 1901), 65.

8. Godias J. Drolit, *Tuberculosis Hospitalization* (New York: New York Tuberculosis and Health Association, 1926), 1–2.

9. Georgina Feldberg, *Disease and Class: Tuberculosis and the Shaping of Modern North American Society* (New Brunswick, N.J.: Rutgers University Press, 1995), 3–4.

10. Matthew Gandy, "Life without Germs: Contested Episodes in the History of Tuberculosis," in Matthew Gandy and Alimuddin Zumla, *The Return of the White Plague: Global Poverty and the "New" Tuberculosis* (New York: Verso, 2003), 18–19.

11. For the story of an upscale sanatorium, where patients dressed for dinner in elaborate evening clothes, see Douglas R. McKay, *Asylum of the Gilded Pill* (Denver: State Historical Society of Colorado, 1983).

12. Billy Jones, *Health Seekers in the Southwest, 1817–1900* (Norman: University of Oklahoma Press, 1967), 7. For an in-depth discussion of the key role tuberculosis played in Colorado specifically, see Jeanne Abrams, *Blazing the Tuberculosis Trail* (Denver: Colorado Historical Society, 1990).

13. See, for example, Gregg Mitman, "Geographies of Hope: Mining the Frontiers of Health in Denver and Beyond, 1870–1965," *Osiris* 19 (2004): 93–111.

14. Thomas Dormandy, *The White Death: A History of Tuberculosis* (New York: New York University Press, 2000), 117.

15. David Rosner, *A Once Charitable Enterprise* (New York: Cambridge University Press, 1982), 12.

16. Charles Rosenberg, *The Care of Strangers: The Rise of America's Hospital System* (New York: Basic Books, 1987), 112.

17. Ibid., 8.

18. Quoted in *First Annual Report of the JCRS, 1905*, 14, JCRS Collection, Box 170, Beck Archives.

19. Emily K. Abel, "Medicine and Morality: The Health Care Program of the New York Charity Organization Society," *Social Service Review* 4 (December 1997): 638.

20. Daniel Ethan Bridge, "The Rise and Development of the Jewish Hospital in America," Rabbinic Ordination Thesis, Hebrew Union College, 1985, 69–130.

21. Kraut, *Silent Travelers,* 225.

22. *The Sanatorium* 1 (March 1907): 1, JCRS Collection, Box 170, Beck Archives.

23. Katherine Ott, *Fevered Lives: Tuberculosis in American Culture since 1870* (Cambridge, Mass.: Harvard University Press, 1996), 148.

24. *The Sanatorium* (May 1907): 49, JCRS Collection, Box 170, Beck Archives.

25. Interview with Ben and Bessie Glass, 1978, Beck Archives.

26. JCRS, *First Annual Report of the JCRS, 1905*, 60, JCRS Collection, Box 167, Beck Archives.

27. Susan Reversby and David Rosner, *Health Care in America* (Philadelphia: Temple University Press, 1979), 1.

28. Charles Spivak to Morris Fred, January 7, 1907, Spivak Biographical File, Beck Archives.

29. Victor Yarros, "Spivak's Early Years," *The Sanatorium* 22 (October–December 1927): 3, JCRS Collection, Box 170, Beck Archives.

30. "Local News: Out of Town—Philadelphia," *The Jewish Messenger,* April 11, 1890, 3.

31. Edward L. Ball, diary transcriber, *The Life of Michael Valentine Ball, 1868–1945* (Warren, Pa.: self-published, 2003), diary entries for April 1 and December 4, 1893, 253, 261.

32. For a more detailed history of National Jewish Hospital, see Mary Ann Fitzharris and Jeanne Abrams, *A Place to Heal: A History of National Jewish Medical and Research Center* (Boulder: Johnson, 1998).

33. Ott, *Fevered Lives,* 94–98.

34. Jeanne Abrams, "Chasing the Cure: A History of the Jewish Consumptives' Relief Society of Denver." Ph.D. diss., University of Colorado at Boulder, 1984, 135, 217.

35. Quoted in *The Sanatorium* 7 (September–December 1914): 95 (Tenth Annual Report), Box 170, Beck Archives.

36. Dr. Charles Spivak to Anna Hillkowitz, May 14, 1906, JCRS Collection, Box 223, Beck Archives.

37. A. Levinson, "Dr. Spivak's Contribution to Medicine," *The Sanatorium* 22 (October–December 1927): 7, JCRS Collection, Box 170, Beck Archives.

38. Interview with Deena Spivak Strauss, March 13, 1982, #90, Oral History Collection, Beck Archives.

39. See, for example, "Correspondence—Spivak," JCRS Collection, Box 222, Beck Archives.

40. *The Forward* (May 28, 1922): 3; *The Forward* (June 25, 1922): 3.

41. Isaac Rivkind, "The Last Days of Dr. Chayim Spivak," *The Sanatorium* 22 (October–December 1927): 12, JCRS Collection, Box 170, Beck Archives.

42. C. E. Hillel Kauvar, "Dr. C. D. Spivak, the Synagogue Jew," *The Sanatorium* 22 (October–December 1927): 9, JCRS Collection, Box 170, Beck Archives.

43. Ball, *Life of Michael Valentine Ball,* diary entry for November 5, 1889, 165.

44. Cited in Harry D. Boonin, *The Jewish Quarter of Philadelphia* (Philadelphia: Jewish Walking Tours of Philadelphia, 1999), 94.

45. Philip Hillkowitz, "Dr. C. D. Spivak and the JCRS," *The Sanatorium* 22 (October–December 1927): 4, JCRS Collection, Box 170, Beck Archives.

46. Boris Bogen, "Dr. Spivak, as Social Worker," *The Sanatorium* 22 (October–December 1927): 7, JCRS Collection, Box 170, Beck Archives.

47. Sheila M. Rothman, *Living in the Shadow of Death: Tuberculosis and the Social Experience of Illness in American History* (New York: Basic Books, 1994), 2.

48. Mark Caldwell, *The Last Crusade: The War on Consumption, 1862–1954* (New York: Atheneum, 1988), 4.

49. For example, physician and historian Frank Ryan, *The Forgotten Plague: How the Battle against Tuberculosis Was Won—and Lost* (Boston: Little, Brown, 1993), 26, claims that despite massive public and private funding, the sanatorium movement "was never subjected to a scientific trial of its effectiveness" and was probably largely unsuccessful in treating patients who were more seriously affected with tuberculosis.

50. Barbara Bates, *Bargaining for Life: A Social History of Tuberculosis, 1876–1938* (Philadelphia: University of Pennsylvania Press, 1992), 318.

51. Gandy, *Return of the White Plague,* 20–27.

52. Alan M. Kraut, "Foreign Bodies: The Perennial Negotiation over Health and Culture in a Nation of Immigrants," *Journal of American Ethnic History* 23 (Winter 2004): 17.

CHAPTER 2: OUT OF RUSSIA

1. There were over 5 million Jews residing in Russia in 1897 and only about 3.5 million in the rest of Europe combined. See "Population," *Encyclopedia Judaica* (Jerusalem: Keter, 1972), 13, 889–892.

2. Steven Cassedy, *To the Other Shore: The Russian Jewish Intellectuals Who Came to America* (Princeton, N.J.: Princeton University Press, 1997), 15.

3. "Biographical Data," *The Sanatorium* 22 (October–December 1927): 2, JCRS Collection, Box 170, and the "Biographical Sketch of Dr. C. D. Spivak,"

Congressional Library at Washington, D.C., Spivak Collection, both in Beck Archives, Special Collections, Penrose Library, University of Denver (hereafter Beck Archives).

4. Benjamin Nathans, *Beyond the Pale: The Jewish Encounter with Late Imperial Russia* (Berkeley: University of California Press, 2002), 218.

5. Ibid., 202; Benjamin Nathans, "The Jews," in Dominic Lieven, ed., *The Cambridge History of Russia, Vol. II, Imperial Russia, 1689–1917* (New York: Cambridge University Press, 2006), 184–202.

6. Harry Boonin, *The Jewish Quarter of Philadelphia* (Philadelphia: Jewish Walking Tours of Philadelphia, 1999), 63–64.

7. Tony Michels, *A Fire in Their Hearts: Yiddish Socialists in New York* (Cambridge, Mass.: Harvard University Press, 2005), 39.

8. Reisen, *Leksikon fun der Yiddisher Literatur Presse un Filologie*, Vol. II, quoted in Jonathan Frankel, *Prophesy and Politics* (New York: Cambridge University Press, 1981), 43.

9. Victor S. Yarros, "Dr. Spivak's Early Days," *The Sanatorium* 22 (October–December 1927): 3, JCRS Collection, Box 170, Beck Archives.

10. Ezra Mendelsohn, "The Russian Roots of the American Jewish Labor Movement," *YIVO Annual of Jewish Social Science* 16 (1976): 152.

11. Yarros, "Dr. Spivak's Early Days," 3.

12. Ibid.

13. Gregory Weinstein, *The Ardent Eighties and After: Reminiscences of a Busy Life* (New York: International Press, 1947), 6.

14. Yarros, "Dr. Spivak's Early Days," 3.

15. Roger Daniels, *Coming to America: A History of Immigration and Ethnicity in American Life* (New York: Harper Perennial, 1991), 224–226.

16. Yarros, "Dr. Spivak's Early Days," 3.

17. Joseph Brandes, *Immigrants to Freedom: Jewish Communities in Rural New Jersey since 1882* (Philadelphia: University of Pennsylvania Press, 1971), 20.

18. Abraham Cahan quoted in "Biographical Data," *The Sanatorium* 22 (October–December 1927): 2, JCRS Collection, Box 170, Beck Archives.

19. Michels, *Fire in Their Hearts*, 21.

20. Gerald Sorin, "Review of *A Fire in Their Hearts*," *American Jewish History* 92 (September 2006): 386.

21. See Rabbi C. E. Hillel Kauvar, "Dr. C. D. Spivak, the Synagogue Jew," *The Sanatorium* 22 (October–December 1927): 9–10, JCRS Collection, Box 170, Beck Archives.

22. Dr. Boris Bogen, "Dr. Spivak, as a Social Worker," *The Sanatorium* 22 (October–December 1927): 5, JCRS Collection, Box 170, Beck Archives.

23. See, for example, Hana Wirth-Nesher's penetrating insights in *Call It English: The Languages of Jewish American Literature* (Princeton, N.J.: Princeton University Press, 2006).

24. Michels, *Fire in Their Hearts*, 53.

25. Ezra Mendelsohn, *Class Struggle in the Pale: The Formative Years of the Jewish Worker's Movement in Tsarist Russia* (London: Cambridge University Press, 1970), viii.

26. Sidney Bailey, "Bailey's Memoirs," in Uri D. Herscher, *Jewish Agricultural Utopias in America* (Detroit: Wayne State University Press, 1981), 149.

27. Abraham Menes, "The Am Olam Movement," *YIVO Annual of Jewish Social Science* 4 (1949): 22.

28. Cited in Frankel, *Prophecy and Politics*, 93.

29. Joel S. Geffen, "Whither: To Palestine or to America in the Pages of the Russian Hebrew Press *Ha-Melitz* and *Ha-Yom* (1880–1890)," *American Jewish Historical Quarterly* 59 (December 1969): 180–181. Dr. Adolph Zederbaum, himself a victim of tuberculosis, later became one of the founders of the JCRS and served as its treasurer alongside Dr. Charles Spivak.

30. Menes, "The Am Olam Movement," 11.

31. Abraham Cahan, *The Education of Abraham Cahan* (Philadelphia: Jewish Publication Society of America, 1969), 182.

32. Alexander Harkavy, "Chapters from My Life," trans. Jonathan Sarna, *American Jewish Archives* 17 (April 1981): 33, 35, 37.

33. Cahan, *Education of Abraham Cahan*, 206.

34. Ibid., 204.

35. Isaac Rivkind, "The Last Days of Dr. Chayim Spivak," *The Sanatorium* 22 (October–December 1927): 13, JCRS Collection, Box 170, Beck Archives.

36. Boris Bogen, *Born a Jew* (New York: Macmillan, 1930), 43.

37. Harkavy, *Chapters from My Life*, 49.

38. Kh. Spivak, "Erinerungen fun Kahan's grine tsaytn," in *Yubeleum-shrift tsu Ab. Kahan's 50stn geburstog* (New York: *The Forward*, 1910), 31–32, quoted in Michels, *Fire in Their Hearts*, 36.

39. Ibid., 39.

40. Dr. H. Schwatt, "The Great Humanitarian," *The Sanatorium* 22 (October–December 1927): 10, JCRS Collection, Box 170, Beck Archives.

41. Gerald Sorin, *The Prophetic Minority: American Jewish Immigrant Radicals, 1880–1920* (Bloomington: Indiana University Press, 1985), 7.

42. Spivak, "Erinerungen fun Kahan's grine tsaytn," 33, quoted in Mendelsohn, "Russian Roots of the American Jewish Labor Movement," 152.

43. "Biographical Sketch of Dr. C. D. Spivak," Congressional Library, Washington, D.C., Spivak Collection, Beck Archives.

44. Quoted in Michels, *Fire in Their Hearts*, 37.

45. I am indebted to Nelly Karmazin, a retired physician born and raised in the Soviet Union, and retired attorney and historian Harry Boonin for their fine English translation from the original Russian.

46. Chaim Spivakovsky, "On the Way in an American Factory," *Voskhod* 21 (1884), reprinted with English translation by Nelly Karmazin and Harry Boonin in *Rocky Mountain Jewish Historical Notes* 16 (Summer-Fall 2001): 2.

47. Ibid.

48. George J. Varney, "History of Lisbon, Maine," in *Gazetteer of the State of Maine* (Boston: B. B. Russell, 1886), 333–336.

49. Spivakovsky, "On the Way in an American Factory," 3.

50. Ibid., 4.

51. Ibid., 5–6.

52. Ibid.

53. Ibid., 7.

54. Ibid.

55. Moses Freeman, *Fuftzig Yohr Geshikhte fun Yidishn Leben in Filadelfia*, Vol. I (Philadelphia: Posy-Shoulson, 1929), 204. Freeman refers to the "Morris" Woolen Mill in his memoir, which was written many years after the event, but no mill by that name is recorded at the Lisbon Falls Library. Freeman may have had a lapse of memory, or he may have known the mill by an informal appellation.

56. Charles Spivak, "Letter to the Editor," *Village News* (Lisbon Falls), reprinted as "Two Letters," *The Sanatorium* 22 (October–December 1927): 18, JCRS Collection, Box 170, Beck Archives.

57. Cassedy, *To the Other Shore*, 106.

58. Spivak, "Letter to the Editor," 18.

59. Cassedy, *To the Other Shore*, xxiii.

60. Sidney Bailey, "Sidney Bailey's Memoirs," in Herscher, *Jewish Agricultural Utopias in America*, 78, 83, 150.

61. Dr. M. Sahud, "Spivak the Modern Saint," *The Sanatorium* 22 (October–December 1927): 11, JCRS Collection, Box 170, Beck Archives.

62. Mendelsohn, "Russian Roots of the American Jewish Labor Movement," 166–167.

63. Brandes, *Immigrants to Freedom*, 93.

64. Spivak letter in *The Jewish Exponent* (Philadelphia), December 27, 1893.

65. Hasia R. Diner, *Hungering for America: Italian, Irish, and Jewish Foodways in the Age of Migration* (Cambridge, Mass.: Harvard University Press, 2001), 12.

66. Werner Sombart, *Why Is There No Socialism in the United States* (White Plains, N.Y.: International Arts and Science Press, 1976 [1906]), 106.

67. Nora Levin, *While Messiah Tarried: The Jewish Socialist Movements, 1871–1917* (New York: Schocken Books, 1977), 179.

68. Cassedy, *To the Other Shore*, 62.

69. Cahan, *Education of Abraham Cahan*, 350.

70. Leon Kobrin, *Mayne Fuftsik Yor in Amerike* (Buenos Aires: Yidbukh bay der Gezelshaft far Yidish-Veltlekhe Shuln in Argentine, 1955), 116.

71. Bogen, "Dr. Spivak, as a Social Worker," 5.

72. Cited in Boonin, *The Jewish Quarter of Philadelphia,* 152.

CHAPTER 3: THE PHILADELPHIA STORY

1. Michael Heilprin was a Polish-born Jewish intellectual and writer who was a strong supporter of the Am Olam movement in the United States and was later active in Jewish relief work. He helped many early Russian immigrants find work in America. When Heilprin died, Spivak organized a memorial meeting in Philadelphia and sent a letter to Reverend Sabato Morais, the spiritual leader of Mikveh Israel, inviting him to join the mourners. He wrote: "Your presence, Reverend Sir, will add to the solemnity of the occasion, and a few words from you, as one who knew him so well would be timely." Letter from Charles Spivak to Rev. Sabato Morais, May 21, 1893, copy on deposit in the Spivak Collection, Beck Archives, Special Collections, Penrose Library, University of Denver (hereafter Beck Archives).

2. Harry Boonin, *The Jewish Quarter of Philadelphia* (Philadelphia: Jewish Walking Tours of Philadelphia, 1999), 20–22. I am grateful to Boonin for both his pathbreaking work on Spivak's life in Philadelphia and his generosity in sharing so many wonderful primary sources he has uncovered.

3. Boris Bogen, "Dr. C. D. Spivak, as a Social Worker," *The Sanatorium* 22 (October–December 1927): 5, JCRS Collection, Box 170, Beck Archives.

4. Edward L. Ball, transcriber, *The Life of Michael Valentine Ball, 1868–1945* (Warren, Pa.: self-published, 2003), diary entry for November 28, 1888, 127.

5. Ibid., diary entry for May 12, 1888, 103.

6. Ibid.

7. Ibid., diary entry for November 10, 1888, 124.

8. Boonin, *Jewish Quarter of Philadelphia*, 63, 77.

9. Ball, *Life of Michael Valentine Ball*, diary entry for September 24, 1887, 79.

10. Ibid., diary entry for November 13, 1887, 83.

11. Ibid., diary entry for November 25, 1888, 127.

12. Ibid., diary entry for November 30, 1888, 128.

13. Victor Yarros, "Spivak's Early Years," *The Sanatorium* 22 (October–December 1927): 3, JCRS Collection, Box 170, Beck Archives.

14. Murray Friedman, ed., *Jewish Life in Philadelphia* (Philadelphia: Jewish Publication Society, 1983), 10.

15. For a thorough discussion of the evolution of medical schools in America, see Kenneth M. Ludmerer, *A Time to Heal: American Medical Education from the Turn of the Century to the Era of Managed Care* (New York: Oxford University Press, 1999), 4–7.

16. Abraham Flexner, *Medical Education in the United States and Canada: A Report to the Carnegie Foundation for the Advancement of Teaching*, Bulletin 4 (New York: Carnegie Foundation, reprint, 1972 [1910]), 111.

17. Ball, *Life of Michael Valentine Ball*, diary entry for November 5, 1889, 165.

18. Boonin, *Jewish Quarter of Philadelphia*, 22.

19. Ball, *Life of Michael Valentine Ball*, diary entry for March 31, 1888, 97.

20. Cited in Boonin, *Jewish Quarter of Philadelphia*, 152.

21. Horeb is an alternate name for Mount Sinai, the mountain on which the Torah, or Five Books of Moses, was given to the Jewish people according to Jewish tradition.

22. Quoted in Jonathan Sarna, *American Judaism* (New Haven: Yale University Press, 2004), 197.

23. *The Jewish Exponent* (Philadelphia), August 24, 1888.

24. Quoted in Boonin, *Jewish Quarter of Philadelphia*, 55.

25. Ball, *Life of Michael Valentine Ball*, diary entry for month of October, 1888, 121.

26. Boonin, *Jewish Quarter of Philadelphia*, 55.

27. A copy of the medical certificate of Dr. Charles Spivak is on deposit in the Spivak Collection, Beck Archives.

28. Letter from Harry Boonin to Jeanne Abrams, January 15, 1995, Spivak Collection, Beck Archives.

29. Ball, *Life of Michael Valentine Ball*, diary entry for April 2, 1890, 193.

30. Ibid., diary entry for April 4, 1890, 193.

31. Ibid.

32. Max Shulman, "Spivak, the Zionist," *The Sanatorium* 22 (October–December 1927): 15, JCRS Collection, Box 170, Beck Archives.

33. Ball, *Life of Michael Valentine Ball*, diary entry for May 22, 1890, 197.

34. Ibid., diary entry for July 1, 1890, 203.

35. Charles E. Rosenberg, "Social Class and Medical Care in 19th-Century America: The Rise and Fall of the Dispensary," in Judith Walzer Leavitt and Ronald L. Numbers, eds., *Sickness and Health in America: Readings in the History of Medicine and Public Health,* 3rd ed. (Madison: University of Wisconsin Press, 1997), 309.

36. Boonin, *Jewish Quarter of Philadelphia*, 82, 63.

37. A. Levinson, M.D., "Dr. Spivak's Contribution to Medicine," *The Sanatorium* 22 (October–December 1927): 7, JCRS Collection, Box 170, Beck Archives.

38. "Writings of Dr. Charles D. Spivak," *The Sanatorium* 11 (October–December 1927): 21, JCRS Collection, Box 170, Beck Archives.

39. *The Philadelphia Inquirer,* August 11, 1890.

40. Charles Spivak to Sabato Morais, August 14, 1890, copy on deposit in the Spivak Collection, Beck Archives.

41. Boonin, *Jewish Quarter of Philadelphia,* 21.

42. Quoted in *The Press* (Philadelphia), August 17, 1891.

43. Quoted in *The Jewish Exponent,* August 29, 1890, 2

44. Ibid., 1.

45. Ibid.

46. Henry Nash Smith, *Virgin Land, the American West as Symbol and Myth* (New York: Vintage Books, 1950), 153.

47. Joseph Brandes, *Immigrants to Freedom: Jewish Communities in Rural New Jersey since 1882* (Philadelphia: University of Pennsylvania Press, 1971), 29–30.

48. Quoted in *The American Israelite,* September 25, 1890, 5.

49. Quoted in *The Jewish Exponent,* August 29, 1887, 7.

50. See, for example, Robert Alter, "The Inner Migration of Hebrew Prose," in David Berger, ed., *The Legacy of Jewish Migration: 1881 and Its Impact* (New York: Brooklyn College Press, 1983).

51. Smith, *Virgin Land*, 183.

52. Quoted in *The Jewish Exponent,* August 29, 1890, 1.

53. Ibid.

54. Hector St. John Crevecoeur, *Letters from an American Farmer* (New York: E. P. Dutton, 1912), 5.

55. *The Jewish Exponent,* December 23, 1887, 1.

56. Quoted in ibid., August 29, 1890, 2.

57. Peter Wiernik, *History of the Jews in America* (New York: Jewish Press Publishing, 1912), 287.

58. *The American Israelite,* February 19, 1891, 2.

59. *The Jewish Exponent*, February 20, 1891, 1.

60. Wiernik, *History of Jews*, 288.

61. *The Public Ledger* (Philadelphia), October 24, 1891.

62. E-mail from Harry Boonin to Jeanne Abrams, November 26, 2006.

63. Leon Kobrin, *Mayne Fuftzig Yor in Amerike* (Buenos Aires: Yidbukh bay der Gezelshaft far Yidish-Veltlekhe Shuln in Argentine, 1955), 116.

64. Ball, *Life of Michael Valentine Ball*, diary entry for August 11, 1892, 243.

65. Ibid., diary entry for February 6, 1893, 250.

66. Ibid., diary entry for February 12, 1893, 251–252.

67. Boonin, *Jewish Quarter of Philadelphia*, 64.

68. Letter from Charles Spivak to Sabato Morais, December 9, 1890, Spivak Collection, Beck Archives.

69. Christine A. Ogren, "A Large Measure of Self-Control and Personal Power: Women Students at State Normal Schools during the Late-Nineteenth and Early-Twentieth Century," *Women's Studies Quarterly* 18 (Fall-Winter 2000): 212–213, 216–217.

70. Boonin, *Jewish Quarter of Philadelphia*, 64, 164.

71. Ball, *Life of Michael Valentine Ball*, diary entry for April 1, 1893, 253.

72. Ibid., 274.

73. Correspondence to Dr. C. D. Spivak, 1922, Mrs. Spivak's Hospitalization Folder, JCRS Collection, Box 222, Beck Archives.

74. Boonin, *Jewish Quarter of Philadelphia*, 64.

75. Ball, *Life of Michael Valentine Ball*, diary entry, July 23, 1893, 157.

76. Ibid., diary entry for August 21, 1893, 258.

77. Ibid., diary entry for December 4, 1893, 261.

78. Ibid.

79. The boarders included Abraham Margolin, a law student at Penn, and Dr. Leo Noy Gartman, who had arrived in America as part of the Am Olam group of which Spivak and Abraham Cahan were members. E-mail from Harry Boonin to Jeanne Abrams, March 20, 2008.

80. Ball, *Life of Michael Valentine Ball,* diary entry for February 25, 1896, 282.

81. Ibid., diary entry for March 5, 1896, 282–283.

82. Ibid., 282.

83. Letter from Charles Spivak to Arnold Kohn, February 27, 1896, copy on deposit in the Spivak Collection, Beck Archives.

84. Cited by Boonin in *Jewish Quarter in Philadelphia*, 74. Boonin garnered the details of the evening from an inscription on the flyleaf of a book of the poems of James Russell Lowell, which was given as a gift to the Spivaks that night.

85. Ball, *Life of Michael Valentine Ball*, diary entry for July 20, 1896, 283.

86. Ibid., 283–284.

87. Ibid.

88. Ibid., diary entry for August 1, 1897, 285.

89. Philip Hillkowitz, "Charles David Spivak, 1861–1927," *The American Review of Tuberculosis* 16 (December 1927): 763–765.

CHAPTER 4: HEADING WEST TO "CHASE THE CURE"

1. Edward Trudeau, *An Autobiography* (New York: Doubleday, Page, 1916), 71.

2. *Tuberculosis in Denver* (Denver: Health Committee of the City Club of Denver, 1925), 5.

3. Renee and Jean Dubois, *The White Plague* (Boston: Little, Brown, 1952), 5.

4. Michael Teller, *The Tuberculosis Movement: A Public Health Campaign in the Progressive Era* (New York: Greenwood, 1988), 17.

5. Trudeau, *An Autobiography*, 29–31.

6. For a clear explanation of the mechanics of the disease, see Barbara Bates, *Bargaining for Life: A Social History of Tuberculosis, 1876–1938* (Philadelphia: University of Pennsylvania Press, 1992), 7; David Barnes, *The Making of a Disease: Tuberculosis in Nineteenth Century France* (Berkeley: University of California Press, 1995), 3.

7. See George Hyde, *Life of George Bent,* ed. Savoie Lottinville (Norman: University of Oklahoma Press, 1962), which reveals that as early as the 1840s the area that became Colorado was beginning to gain a reputation for healthfulness.

8. Denver Chamber of Commerce, *Fourth Annual Report* (Denver: Denver Chamber of Commerce, 1887), 56.

9. *The Heart of the Rockies* (Denver: Denver & Rio Grande Railroad, 1880), 22.

10. E. R. Axtell, "Tent Life for Consumptives," *The Colorado Climatologist* 1 (May 1895): 160.

11. Thomas Galbreath, *Chasing the Cure in Colorado* (Denver: self-published, 1907), 40.

12. James Giese, "Tuberculosis and the Growth of Denver's Eastern European Jewish Community: The Accommodation of an Immigrant Group to a Medium-Sized Western City, 1900–1920," Ph.D. diss., University of Colorado, 1979, 11.

13. Billy Jones, *Health Seekers in the Southwest, 1817–1900* (Norman: University of Oklahoma Press, 1967), 89.

14. Galbreath, *Chasing the Cure in Colorado*, 20.

15. Interview with Deena Spivak Strauss, March 13, 1982, #90, Oral History Collection, Beck Archives, Special Collections, Penrose Library, University of Denver (hereafter Beck Archives).

16. A. J. Magruder, "Physicians in Colorado for Tuberculosis," *Denver Medical Times* 28 (October 1908): 152.

17. Cited in Fred Harper, *The Story of Tuberculosis and the Evangelical Lutheran Sanitarium* (Denver: Lutheran Hospital, 1980), 7.

18. Charles Denison, "How Does Climate Influence Tuberculosis?" *Denver Medical Times* 28 (1908): 141–144.

19. Luther H. Woods, "Seeking Health in Colorado," *Denver Medical Times* 18 (May 1899): 535.

20. Quoted in Bates, *Bargaining for Life*, 28.

21. Thomas Galbreath, *T.B.: Playing the Lone Game Consumption* (New York: Journal of the Outdoor Life, 1915), 49.

22. Alice Boggs, "The History and Development of the Tuberculosis Assistance Program in Colorado," M.A. thesis, University of Denver, 1943, 1.

23. Jacob Chester Teller, *Report on the Problem of Combined Poverty and Tuberculosis in Denver, Colorado* (New York: National Conference of Jewish Charities, 1916), 30.

24. Sherman Bonney, "What Consumptives Should Come to Colorado?" *Denver Medical Times* 28 (October 1908): 146.

25. Emily K. Abel, "Medicine and Morality: The Health Care Program of the New York Charity Organization Society," *Social Service Review* 71 (December 1997): 638.

26. Ibid., 637.

27. Cited in Bates, *Bargaining for Life*, 58.

28. Teller, *Tuberculosis Movement*, 21.

29. Gunther Barth, *Instant Cities: Urbanization and the Rise of San Francisco and Denver* (New York: Oxford University Press, 1975), 129, 136, 138.

30. Cited in Allen Breck, *A Centennial History of the Jews of Colorado* (Denver: Hirschfeld, 1960), 321.

31. Marjorie Hornbein, "Frances Jacobs: Denver's Mother of Charities," *Western States Jewish Historical Quarterly* 14 (January 1983): 131–133. For a fuller discussion of the life and times of Frances Jacobs, see Jeanne Abrams, *Jewish Women Pioneering the Frontier Trail: A History in the American West* (New York: New York University Press, 2006).

32. For a general discussion of the subject of "women's sphere," see Linda Kerber, "Separate Spheres, Female Worlds, Woman's Place: The Rhetoric of Women's History," *The Journal of American History* 75 (June 1988): 9–39.

33. Hornbein, "Frances Jacobs," 131–133; *Memoirs of Frances Jacobs* (Denver: Charity Organization Society, 1892); Abrams, *Jewish Women Pioneering the Frontier Trail*, 51–54.

34. Hornbein, "Frances Jacobs," 140–143.

35. Henry Berkowitz to Charles Spivak, June 11, 1897, and Charles Spivak to Denver NCJW, June 18, 1897, both in JCRS Collection, Box 222, Beck Archives.

36. For a detailed history of the NCJW, see Faith Rogow, *Gone to Another Meeting: The National Council of Jewish Women, 1890–1993* (Tuscaloosa: University of Alabama Press, 1993).

37. Charles Spivak to Charles Hoffman, July 9, 1897, Spivak Correspondence Folder, JCRS Collection, Box 222, Beck Archives.

38. *The Denver Times,* December 17, 1899.

39. NJH, *First Annual Report for 1900*, 64, NJH Collection, Box 31, Beck Archives.

40. Dr. M. Sahud, "Spivak, the Modern Saint," *The Sanatorium* 22 (October–December 1927): 11, JCRS Collection, Box 170, Beck Archives.

41. Ibid.

42. Charles Spivak to Mayer Sulzberger, December 13, 1904, Spivak Collection, Beck Archives.

43. "Biographical Sketch of Dr. C. D. Spivak," The Congressional Library at Washington, D.C., 1, Spivak Collection, Beck Archives.

44. Sahud, "Spivak, the Modern Saint," 12.

45. Dr. A. Levinson, "Dr. Spivak's Contribution to Medicine," *The Sanatorium* 22 (October–December 1927): 7–8, JCRS Collection, Box 170, Beck Archives.

46. "Biographical Sketch of Dr. C. D. Spivak," 1.

47. Dr. Charles Spivak, "Rest—A Neglected Factor in the Treatment of Gastro-Intestinal Disorder," *Journal of the American Medical Association* 21 (July 30, 1898): 216.

48. For a complete list of Spivak's published work, see "Writings of Dr. Charles D. Spivak," *The Sanatorium* 22 (October–December 1927): 21–23, JCRS Collection, Box 170, Beck Archives.

49. Ibid., 21; Philip Hillkowitz, "Charles David Spivak, 1861–1927," *The American Review of Tuberculosis* 16 (December 1927): 763.

50. *Medical Life,* January 1928.

51. C. D. Spivak, "The Union Catalogue of Medical Books, and Some of the Private Medical Libraries in the City of Denver," *The Colorado Medical Journal* 3 (1897): 214.

52. Francis Tandy, "The Colorado Medical Library Association," *Medical Libraries* 1 (May 1898): 27.

53. *Journal of the American Medical Association* (January 22, 1898), quoted in Levinson, "Dr. Spivak's Contribution to Medicine," 8.

54. C. Spivak, "Medical Reprints," *Journal of the American Medical Association* 39 (1902): 1018.

55. *Medical Libraries* 1 (February 1898): 1 (quote), and 1 (May 1898): 30.

56. *Medical Libraries* 2 (January 1899): 57; C. D. Spivak, "The Medical Libraries of the United States," *Medical Libraries Supplement* (January 1899): 1.

57. Earl Pomeroy, "On Becoming a Westerner," in Moses Rischin and John Livingston, eds., *Jews of the American West* (Detroit: Wayne State University Press, 1991), 202.

58. Ibid., 196–197.

59. Ferenc Morton Szasz, *Religion in the Modern American West* (Tucson: University of Arizona Press, 2000), xii, xvi.

60. For a fine study of women's suffrage in the American West, see Rebecca Mead, *How the Vote Was Won* (New York: New York University Press, 2004).

61. *University of Denver Bulletins*, 1903–1913, Special Collections, Penrose Library, University of Denver.

62. Ida Uchill, *Pioneers, Peddlers, and Tsadikim* (Denver: Sage, 1959), 158.

63. Naomi Cohen, *Encounter with Emancipation* (Philadelphia: Jewish Publication Society, 1984), 114, 117.

64. Quoted in Milton Anfenger, *The Birth of a Hospital: The Story of the Birth of the National Jewish Hospital in Denver* (Denver: National Jewish Hospital, 1943), 15–16.

65. Abraham Karp, *Golden Door to America: The Jewish Immigrant Experience* (New York: Viking, 1976), 14.

66. Boris D. Bogen, *Born a Jew* (New York: Macmillan, 1930), 60.

67. *Jewish Outlook* (Denver), October 7, 1904.

68. Alan M. Kraut, *Silent Travelers: Germs, Genes, and the "Immigrant Menace"* (New York: Basic Books, 1994), 2.

69. National Jewish Hospital, *First Annual Report, 1900*, 17, NJH Collection, Box 31, Beck Archives.

70. Teller, *Tuberculosis Movement*, 26.

71. Bates, *Bargaining for Life*, 180.

72. Georgina D. Feldberg, *Disease and Class: Tuberculosis and the Shaping of Modern North American Society* (New Brunswick, N.J.: Rutgers University Press, 1995), 92.

73. Cited in NJH, *First Annual Report*, 5.

74. Dr. Boris Bogen, "Dr. Spivak as a Social Worker," *The Sanatorium* 22 (October–December 1927): 5, JCRS Collection, Box 170, Beck Archives.

75. Hillkowitz, "Charles David Spivak, 1861–1927," 765.

76. Dr. C. D. Spivak, "Pulmonary Tuberculosis, the Care of Advanced Cases—A Plea for Scientific, Practical and Humane Methods of Eradicating the White Plague," *The Sanatorium* 1 (May 1907): 65–66, JCRS Collection, Box 170, Beck Archives.

77. Cited in *The Denver Jewish News*, April 1925, 10.

78. Boris Bogen, *Jewish Philanthropy* (New York: Macmillan, 1917), x.

79. B'nai B'rith of Denver, Minutes, 5 (April 9, 1905), 115, and 5 (April 23, 1905), 122, B'nai B'rith Collection, Beck Archives.

80. In their unpublished essay (Rosslyn Stewart and Laurie Simmons, "A Small Gathering of Men: The Origins of Denver's Jewish Consumptives' Relief Society,"

November 1981), the authors speculate that Spivak's rejection by the Denver B'nai B'rith may have been a general rejection by the German Jewish community, which might have prompted him to support the JCRS. However, Spivak's association with the JCRS dates back to 1903, well before his 1905 membership refusal by the B'nai B'rith.

81. Teller, *Report on the Problem of Combined Poverty and Tuberculosis*, 5.

82. Ibid.

83. B'nai B'rith, Minutes 28 (June 1908), 174.

84. Interview with Deena Spivak Strauss, March 13, 1982, #90, Oral History Collection, Beck Archives.

85. "Dr. C. D. Spivak and the JCRS," *The Sanatorium* 22 (October–December 1927): 4, JCRS Collection, Box 170, Beck Archives.

CHAPTER 5: THE GENESIS OF THE JCRS: CREATING A NEW TYPE OF TB INSTITUTION

1. Dr. Charles Spivak, "Secretary's Report," *First Annual Report of the JCRS, 1905*, 23, JCRS Collection, Box 170, Beck Archives, Special Collections, Penrose Library, University of Denver (hereafter Beck Archives).

2. Dr. Philip Hillkowitz, "President's Report," *First Annual Report of the JCRS, 1905*, 12, Beck Archives.

3. Quoted in Barbara Bates, *Bargaining for Life: A Social History of Tuberculosis, 1876–1938* (Philadelphia: University of Pennsylvania Press, 1992), 1, 58.

4. "Editorial," *The Sanatorium* 4 (November–December 1910): 208, JCRS Collection, Box 170, Beck Archives.

5. *First Annual Report of the JCRS, 1905*, 3, 27.

6. JCRS Board of Trustees Minutes, Book #1, July 30, 1904, 64, JCRS Collection, Box 298, Beck Archives.

7. Spivak, "Secretary's Report," *First Annual Report of the JCRS, 1905*, 29.

8. JCRS Board of Trustees Minutes, Book #8, July 18, 1917, 7, JCRS Collection, Box 298, Beck Archives.

9. *The Denver Republican,* August 2, 1904.

10. JCRS Board of Trustees Minutes, February 9, 1921, JCRS Collection, Box 298, Beck Archives.

11. Hillkowitz Biographical File, Beck Archives.

12. Author's conversation with Ben Glass, August 2, 1983, Denver.

13. "Editorial," *The Sanatorium* 3 (September–October 1909): 253, JCRS Collection, Box 170, Beck Archives.

14. "Seder Service," *The Sanatorium* 1 (May 1906): 55, JCRS Collection, Box 170, Beck Archives.

15. Hasia R. Diner, *Hungering for America: Italian, Irish, and Jewish Foodways in the Age of Migration* (Cambridge, Mass.: Harvard University Press, 2001), 8.

16. Leon Kobrin, *A Lithuanian Village* (New York: Bernard G. Richards, 1927).

17. "Secretary's Report," *Sixth Annual Report, The Sanatorium* 4 (March–June 1910): 47, JCRS Collection, Box 170, Beck Archives.

18. Georgina Feldberg, *Disease and Class: Tuberculosis and the Shaping of Modern North American Society* (New Brunswick, N.J.: Rutgers University Press, 1995), 82.

19. See, for example, overview in Judith Walzer Leavitt and Ronald L. Numbers, eds., *Sickness and Health in America: Readings in the History of Medicine and Public Health,* 3rd ed. (Madison: University of Wisconsin Press, 1997), 3–10.

20. Nancy Tomes, *The Gospel of Germs: Men, Women, and the Microbe in American Life* (Cambridge, Mass.: Harvard University Press, 1988), 18.

21. Ibid., 124.

22. "Stereopticon Views on Consumption," *The Sanatorium* 1 (September 1907): 166, JCRS Collection, Box 170, Beck Archives.

23. Feldberg, *Disease and Class*, 122.

24. M. J. Rosenau, E. C. Schroeder, and Emile Berliner, "Simple Lessons on Tuberculosis or Consumption," *The Sanatorium* 3 (January 1909): 23–24, JCRS Collection, Box 170, Beck Archives.

25. Charles Spivak, "Don't Crawl into a Clean Bed with Dirty Feet," *The Forward,* June 25, 1922.

26. C. D. Spivak, "The Genesis and Growth of the Jewish Consumptives Relief Society. I," *The Sanatorium* 1 (January 1907): 5, JCRS Collection, Box 170, Beck Archives.

27. Dr. Boris Bogen, "Dr. Spivak, as a Social Worker," *The Sanatorium* 22 (October–December 1927): 5, JCRS Collection, Box 170, Beck Archives.

28. *Jewish Outlook* (Denver), April 15, 1904, 7–8.

29. Bogen, "Dr. Spivak, as a Social Worker," 6.

30. Quoted in *Second Annual Report of the JCRS, 1906,* 11, JCRS Collection, Box 170, Beck Archives.

31. For example, see David Filene, "An Obituary for the 'Progressive Movement,'" *American Quarterly* 22 (Spring 1970): 20–34; John Burnham, "Essay," in John D. Buenker, John C. Burnham, and Robert M. Cruden, eds., *Progressivism* (Cambridge, Mass.: Harvard University Press, 1977), 31–69.

32. "Editorial," *The Sanatorium* 1 (May 1907): 41, JCRS Collection, Box 170, Beck Archives.

33. "Secretary's Report for 1906," *The Sanatorium* 1 (July 1907): 90–91, JCRS Collection, Box 170, Beck Archives.

34. Patient Records, JCRS Collection, Box 97, Beck Archives.

35. Interview with Deena Spivak Strauss, March 13, 1982, #90, Oral History Collection, Beck Archives.

36. JCRS Board of Trustees Minutes, 1903–1924, JCRS Collection, Box 298, Beck Archives.

37. *The Sanatorium* 1 (May 1907): 55, JCRS Collection, Box 170, Beck Archives.

38. Cited in *The Sanatorium* 1 (November 1907): 193, JCRS Collection, Box 170, Beck Archives.

39. Dr. Philip Hillkowitz, "Dr. C. D. Spivak and the JCRS," *The Sanatorium* 22 (October–December 1927): 5, JCRS Collection, Box 170, Beck Archives.

40. Tomes, *Gospel of Germs*, 117.

41. Chester Jacob Teller, *Report on the Combined Problem of Tuberculosis and Poverty among Jews in Denver* (New York: National Conference of Jewish Charities, 1916), 93.

42. The many boxes in the JCRS Collection contain countless receipts and general correspondence that acknowledge small contributions. In particular, Boxes 233–235 and the JCRS Book of Life, Boxes, 269–293, record literally thousands of modest contributions.

43. JCRS Board of Trustees Minutes, October 11, 1904, JCRS Collection, Box 298, Beck Archives.

44. Letter from Spivak to Hillkowitz, May 14, 1906, JCRS Collection, Box 223, Beck Archives.

45. Letter from Spivak to Hillkowitz, January 13, 1906, JCRS Collection, Box 223, Beck Archives.

46. Letter from Spivak to Hillkowitz, December 29, 1906, JCRS Collection, Box 223, Beck Archives.

47. Letter from Spivak to Hillkowitz, April 12, 1906, and letter from Spivak to Hillkowitz, September 28, 1906, both in JCRS Collection, Box 223, Beck Archives.

48. *The Sanatorium* 1 (November 1907): 203, JCRS Collection, Box 170, Beck Archives.

49. *The Sanatorium* 1 (January 1907): 33, JCRS Collection, Box 170, Beck Archives.

50. See *First Annual Report of the JCRS, 1905; Second Annual Report of the JCRS, 1906*; and *The Sanatorium*, 1907–1927, all in JCRS Collection, Box 170, Beck Archives.

51. Feldberg, *Disease and Class*, 52.

52. Spivak, "Secretary's Report," *First Annual Report of the JCRS, 1905*, 32.

53. Ernest Poole, "The Lung Block," in Robert Bremner, *Children and Youth in America: A Documentary History*, Vol. II: *1866–1923* (Cambridge, Mass.: Harvard University Press, 1971 [1903]), 886–887.

54. Hillkowitz, "President's Address," *Second Annual Report of the JCRS, 1906*, 12.

55. "The Medical Department of the J.C.R.S.," *The Sanatorium* 2 (September 1908): 240–241, JCRS Collection, Box 170, Beck Archives.

56. Spivak, "Secretary's Report," *The Sanatorium* 5 (May–August 1911): 109, JCRS Collection, Box 170, Beck Archives.

57. Renee and Jean Dubois, *The White Plague: Man and Society* (Boston: Little, Brown, 1952), 173; Mark Caldwell, *The Last Crusade: The War on Consumption, 1862–1954* (New York: Athenuem, 1988), 10, 180.

58. Spivak, "Secretary's Report," *First Annual Report of the JCRS, 1905,* 60, 31.

59. Hillkowitz, "President's Address," *First Annual Report of the JCRS, 1905*, 14.

60. Dr. Adolph Zederbaum, "Kosher Meat in Jewish Hospitals and Sanatoria," *The Sanatorium* 2 (November 1908): 275, JCRS Collection, Box 170, Beck Archives.

61. Hillkowitz, "President's Address," *First Annual Report of the JCRS, 1905*, 14.

62. Douglas R. McKay, "A History of the Nordrach Ranch: Colorado's First Sanatorium of the Open Air," *The Colorado Magazine* 56 (Summer-Fall 1979): 184–185.

63. Feldberg, *Disease and Class*, 53.

64. Quoted in Thomas M. Daniel, *Captain of Death: The Story of Tuberculosis* (Rochester, N.Y.: University of Rochester Press, 1999), 189.

65. "Leon Kobrin's Drama," *The Sanatorium* 2 (May 1908): 130, JCRS Collection, Box 170, Beck Archives.

66. *The Sanatorium* 5 (January–February 1911): 31, JCRS Collection, Box 170, Beck Archives.

67. Interview with Deena Spivak Strauss, March 13, 1982, #90, Oral History Collection, Beck Archives. In 1891 Alexander Harkavy, Spivak's fellow Russian immigrant, first published a highly regarded Yiddish-English-Hebrew dictionary, which has been reprinted many times. Its continuing popularity is probably a result of the fact that unlike Spivak's work, Harkavy's incorporated English and Hebrew.

68. *The Intermountain Jewish News* (Denver), May 19, 1920, 1.

69. "The Yehoash Receptions," *The Sanatorium* 2 (November 1908): 285, JCRS Collection, Box 170, Beck Archives.

70. *First Annual Report of the JCRS, 1905.*

71. Jacob Marinoff to Dr. Spivak, December 12, 1913, JCRS Collection, Box 222, Beck Archives (original emphasis).

72. Hillkowitz, "President's Address," *First Annual Report of the JCRS, 1905,* 13.

73. C. D. Spivak, "The Genesis and Growth of the Jewish Consumptives Relief Society, IV," *The Sanatorium* 1 (September 1907): 139, JCRS Collection, Box 170, Beck Archives.

74. Cited in Sheila M. Rothman, *Living in the Shadow of Death: Tuberculosis and the Social Experience of Illness in American History* (New York: Basic Books, 1994), 6.

75. Spivak, "Secretary's Report," *First Annual Report of the JCRS, 1905*, 29.

76. Unidentified, undated newspaper clipping on Simpkins, JCRS Scrapbook no. 1, JCRS Collection, Box 197, Beck Archives.

77. Spivak, "Secretary's Report," *Second Annual Report of the JCRS, 1906,* 25.

78. Frank Ryan, *The Forgotten Plague: How the Battle against Tuberculosis Was Won—and Lost* (Boston: Little, Brown, 1993), 28.

79. Katherine Ott, *Fevered Lives: Tuberculosis in American Culture since 1870* (Cambridge, Mass.: Harvard University Press, 1996), 97–99.

80. Bates, *Bargaining for Life*, 286.

81. *45th Annual Medical Report of the JCRS*, 1948, 3, JCRS Collection, Box 255, Beck Archives.

82. Interview with Deena Spivak Strauss, March 13, 1982, #90, Oral History Collection, Beck Archives.

83. Cited in Marjorie Hornbein, "Dr. Charles Spivak of Denver: Physician, Social Worker, Yiddish Author," *Western States Jewish Historical Quarterly* 11 (April 1977): 195.

84. Interview with Deena Spivak Strauss, March 13, 1982, Beck Archives.

85. Spivak, "Secretary's Report," *First Annual Report of the JCRS, 1905*, 35.

86. Interview with Deena Spivak Strauss, March 13, 1982, Beck Archives.

87. Interview with Adele Strauss Karsh conducted by Susan Goldman, May 29, 2005, Beck Archives.

88. Rabbi C. E. Hillel Kauvar, "Dr. C. D. Spivak, the Synagogue Jew," *The Sanatorium* 22 (September–December 1927): 9, JCRS Collection, Box 170, Beck Archives.

89. Gregory Weinstein, *The Ardent Eighties and After: Reminiscences of a Busy Life* (New York: International Press, 1947), 3.

90. Cited in JCRS Board of Trustees Minutes, June 8, 1909, JCRS Collection, Box 298, Beck Archives.

91. Ida Uchill, *Pioneers, Peddlers, and Tsadikim* (Denver: Sage, 1959), 255.

92. Kauvar, "Dr. C. D. Spivak, the Synagogue Jew," 10.

93. Ibid.

94. Quoted in Joseph Brandes, *Immigrants to Freedom; Jewish Communities in Rural New Jersey since 1882* (Philadelphia: University of Pennsylvania Press, 1971), 215.

95. Edward L. Ball, diary transcriber, *The Life of Michael Valentine Ball, 1868–1945* (Warren, Pa.: self-published, 2003), diary entry for April 1, 1893, 253.

96. *The Jewish Exponent*, August 18, 1899.

97. *The Sanatorium* 2 (September 1908): 241, JCRS Collection, Box 170, Beck Archives.

98. "Editorial," *The Sanatorium* 3 (January 1909): 1, JCRS Collection, Box 170, Beck Archives.

CHAPTER 6: BECOMING A WESTERNER

1. For Jewish population trends in early Denver, see Appendix A, in Allen Breck, *A Centennial History of the Jews of Colorado* (Denver: Hirschfeld, 1960), 321.

2. Dr. Charles Spivak, "The Tenth Annual Report of the JCRS," *The Sanatorium* 13 (September–December 1914): 93–94, JCRS Collection, Box 170, Beck Archives, Special Collections, Penrose Library, University of Denver (hereafter Beck Archives).

3. Minutes, JCRS Executive Committee, April 25, 1911, Minute Book 5, JCRS Collection, Box 298, Beck Archives.

4. Breck, *Centennial History of the Jews of Colorado*, 110–111, 191.

5. Quoted in *The Intermountain Jewish News* (Denver), March 26, 1953, 12.

6. C. D. Spivak, "The Jews of West Colfax," *The Denver Jewish News*, March 12, 1915, 10.

7. Dr. Charles Spivak, "Post Mortem Examinations among the Jews—An Historical Sketch and a Plea to Jewish Physicians," *New York Journal of Medicine* (June 13, 1914): 1185.

8. Alan Kraut, *Silent Travelers: Germs, Genes, and the "Immigrant Menace"* (New York: Basic Books, 1994), 148–149. Spivak and Fishberg were articulate advocates for East European Jewish immigrants and exceptional examples of Jewish physicians who served as "ethnic brokers" or "cultural mediators."

9. C. D. Spivak, "Why Jews Are Not Prohibitionists," *The Denver Jewish News*, January 7, 1916, 1–2.

10. C. D. Spivak, "Rabbi Hirschberg He Does Not Like Yiddish," *The Denver Jewish News*, May 5, 1916, 140.

11. "Writings of Dr. Charles D. Spivak," *The Sanatorium* 22 (October–December 1927): 22, JCRS Collection, Box 170, Beck Archives.

12. Ida Uchill, *Pioneers, Peddlers, and Tsadkim* (Denver: Sage, 1959), 257.

13. Alfred W. Pick to Dr. C. D. Spivak, October 6, 1921, JCRS Collection, Box 222, Beck Archives.

14. Dr. C. D. Spivak, "The Jewish Physicians of Colorado, Biographic and Bibliographic," unpublished manuscript, Spivak Collection, Beck Archives, and "Contributions of Colorado Jewish Physicians to Medical Literature," *The Denver Jewish News* July 24, 1924, 10.

15. Quoted in *The Sanatorium* 11 (January–March 1917): 7–9, JCRS Collection, Box 222, Beck Archives (original emphasis).

16. Spivak, "Tenth Annual Report," 96.

17. Dr. Philip Hillkowitz, "President's Address," *The JCRS Bulletin* 1 (January–February 1931): 2–3, JCRS Collection, Box 255, Beck Archives.

18. Dr. Charles Spivak, "Secretary's Report, Seventh Annual Report of the JCRS," *The Sanatorium* 10 (September–December 1911): 114, JCRS Collection, Box 170, Beck Archives.

19. Dr. Herman Schwatt, "Superintendent's Report, Tenth Annual Report of the JCRS," *The Sanatorium* 8 (September–December 1914): 98, JCRS Collection, Box 170, Beck Archives.

20. Quoted in JCRS Board of Trustees Minutes, Book 8, July 18, 1917, 7, JCRS Collection, Box 298, Beck Archives.

21. David Rosner, *A Once Charitable Enterprise* (New York: Cambridge University Press, 1982), 1, 19.

22. Ibid., 108.

23. Jacob Lindenthal, "Abi Gezunt: Health and the Eastern European Jewish Immigrant," *American Jewish History* 70 (June 1981): 440–442; Kraut, *Silent Travelers*, 141.

24. Chester Jacob Teller, *Report on the Problem of Combined Poverty and Tuberculosis among Jews in Denver, Colorado* (New York: National Conference of Jewish Charities, 1916), 107.

25. Cited in *The Sanatorium* 22 (April–June 1927): 54, JCRS Collection, Box 170, Beck Archives.

26. Interview with Adele Strauss Karsh conducted by Susan Goldman, May 29, 2005, Beck Archives.

27. Alan M. Kraut, "Foreign Bodies: The Perennial Negotiation over Health and Culture in a Nation of Immigrants," *Journal of American Ethnic History* 23 (Winter 2004): 8–10.

28. Minutes of the JCRS Trustees, July 19, 1911, JCRS Collection, Box 298, Beck Archives.

29. C. D. Spivak, M.D., "The Mortality of the Jews in Denver," *The Sanatorium* 18 (January–March 1924): 6, JCRS Collection, Box 170, Beck Archives.

30. Philip Hillkowitz, "Charles David Spivak, 1861–1927," *The American Review of Tuberculosis* 16 (December 1927): 763.

31. Dr. C. D. Spivak, "Meeting the Problem of the Indigent Tuberculous among the Jews," *The Sanatorium* 13 (January–March 1919): 3, JCRS Collection, Box 222, Beck Archives.

32. Teller, *Report on the Problem of Combined Poverty and Tuberculosis*, 100.

33. Dr. A. Levinson, "Dr. Chayim Spivak, an Appreciation," *The Chicago Chronicle*, October 28, 1927, clipping, Spivak Memorial Scrapbook, JCRS Collection, Box 222, Beck Archives.

34. Spivak to Dr. Michael Ball, March 2, 1907, Dr. Charles Spivak Collection, Beck Archives.

35. Interview with Deena Spivak Strauss, March 13, 1983, #90, Oral History Collection, Beck Archives.

36. Ibid.

37. Spivak to Max Maisel, February 12, 1912, JCRS Collection, Box 222, Beck Archives.

38. "Editorial," *The Sanatorium* 5 (January–February 1911): 3–4, JCRS Collection, Box 222, Beck Archives.

39. C. D. Spivak, "Hatikvah—A Publication of Hope," *The Sanatorium* 17 (January–March 1923): 6, JCRS Collection, Box 170, Beck Archives.

40. See Alan Kraut, *Goldberger's War: The Life and Work of a Public Health Crusader* (New York: Hill and Wang, 2003).

41. Interview with Deena Spivak Strauss, March 13, 1983, #90, Oral History Collection, Beck Archives.

42. Ibid.

43. *The Sanatorium* 9 (January–February 1915): 14, JCRS Collection, Box 222, Beck Archives.

44. Deena Spivak to Charles Spivak, June 23, 1915, JCRS Collection, Box 223, Beck Archives.

45. Ruth Spivak to Charles Spivak, June 24, 1915, JCRS Collection, Box 222, Beck Archives.

46. Ruth and Deena Spivak to Charles and Jennie Spivak, August 24, 1915, JCRS Collection, Box 222, Beck Archives.

47. Michael Zelinger, *West Side Story Relived* (Denver: Wandel, 1987), 93.

48. *Denver City Directory* (Denver: Gazetteer, 1923, 1927).

49. Undated letter, Deena Spivak to Charles Spivak, JCRS Collection, Box 222, Beck Archives.

50. Deena Spivak to Charles and Ruth Spivak, August 9, 1915, JCRS Collection, Box 222, Beck Archives.

51. Deena Spivak to Charles and Ruth Spivak, September 28, 1915, JCRS Collection, Box 222, Beck Archives.

52. Undated letter, Deena Spivak to Charles Spivak, JCRS Collection, Box 222, Beck Archives.

53. Deena Spivak to Charles Spivak, December 6, 1915, JCRS Collection, Box 222, Beck Archives.

54. Postcard from Deena Spivak to Charles Spivak, December 2, 1916, JCRS Collection, Box 222, Beck Archives.

55. Deena Spivak to Charles Spivak, December 4, 1916, JCRS Collection, Box 222, Beck Archives.

56. Deena Spivak to Spivak family, January 4, 1916 (Norfolk), JCRS Collection, Box 222, Beck Archives.

57. Deena Spivak to Ruth, Jennie, and Charles Spivak, January 30, 1917, JCRS Collection, Box 222, Beck Archives (original emphasis).

58. Undated letter, Deena Spivak to Charles Spivak, JCRS Collection, Box 222, Beck Archives.

59. Interview with Deena Spivak Strauss, March 13, 1983, #90, Oral History Collection, Beck Archives.

60. Uchill, *Pioneers, Peddlers, and Tsadikim*, 258.

61. *Denver City Directory* (Denver: Gazetteer, 1912).

62. Edward Ball, diary transcriber, *The Life of Michael Valentine Ball, 1868–1945* (Warren, Pa.: self-published, 2003), diary entry for May 1917, 397.

63. David Spivak to Charles Spivak, November 14, 1915, JCRS Collection, Box 222, Beck Archives.

64. David Spivak to Ruth Spivak, December 2, 1915, JCRS Collection, Box 222, Beck Archives.

65. Jennie Spivak to Ruth Spivak, May 26, 1916, JCRS Collection, Box 222, Beck Archives.

66. Undated letter, Deena Spivak to David Spivak, JCRS Collection, Box 222, Beck Archives (original emphasis).

67. Ibid.

68. *Denver City Directory* (Denver: Gazetteer: 1918, 1919).

69. Undated letter, Ruth Spivak to Charles Spivak, JCRS Collection, Box 222, Beck Archives.

70. David Spivak to Charles Spivak, July 14, 1921, JCRS Collection, Box 222, Beck Archives.

71. *Denver City Directory* (Denver: Gazetteer: 1923).

72. David Spivak to Charles Spivak, May 26, 1925, JCRS Collection, Box 222, Beck Archives.

73. David Spivak to Lee Frankel, July 9, 1929, and Lee Frankel to David Spivak, July 16, 1929, Lee K. Frankel Papers, American Jewish Historical Society, New York City.

74. *David Spivak—Catalog of Paintings, 1914–1932* (Denver: Denver Art Museum, 1932), 1–8, Photo Collection #530, Beck Archives.

75. Ibid., 9.

CHAPTER 7: MISSION OVERSEAS TO THE EUROPEAN FRONT AND THE FINAL YEARS

1. Arthur Hertzberg, *The Jews in America* (New York: Simon and Schuster, 1989), 226, 236.

2. Naomi Cohen, *Not Free to Desist* (Philadelphia: Jewish Publication Society, 1972), 120.

3. "The Gift of the JCRS to the War Sufferers," *The Sanatorium* 14 (January–March 1920): 3, JCRS Collection, Box 170, Beck Archives, Special Collections, Penrose Library, University of Denver (hereafter Beck Archives).

4. Ibid., 4.

5. Spivak Testimonial Dinner Booklet, December 28, 1919, Spivak Biographical File, Beck Archives.

6. "Dr. C. D. Spivak Honored Guest at Banquet and Reception Given by Denver Jewry," *The Sanatorium* 14 (January–March 1920): 5–6, JCRS Collection, Box 170, Beck Archives.

7. Boris D. Bogen, *Born a Jew* (New York: Macmillan, 1930), 219–220.

8. Dr. Boris D. Bogen, "Dr. Spivak, as a Social Worker," *The Sanatorium* 22 (October–December 1927): 6, JCRS Collection, Box 170, Beck Archives.

9. Ibid., 6–7.

10. *The Sanatorium* 6 (July–October 1912): 99, JCRS Collection, Box 170, Beck Archives.

11. Quoted in *The Denver Jewish News,* March 26, 1953, 12.

12. Ibid., May 19, 1920, 1.

13. Ibid.

14. "Confidential Report Dated Warsaw, April 13, 1920 from Dr. Spivak," 1, copy on deposit in the JCRS Collection, Box 222, Beck Archives.

15. Ibid., 2–5.

16. Ibid., 6–10.

17. Ibid., 11–12.

18. Ibid., 13–19.

19. David Glassberg, "The Design of Reform: The Public Bath Movement in America," in Judith Walzer Leavitt and Ronald L. Numbers, eds., *Sickness and Health in America: Readings in the History of Medicine and Public Health,* 3rd ed. (Madison: University of Wisconsin Press, 1997), 485–488.

20. Ida Uchill, *Pioneers, Peddlers, and Tsadikim* (Denver: Sage, 1959), 253.

21. "Dr. Spivak in War-Torn Europe," *The Sanatorium* 14 (April–June 1920): 23, JCRS Collection, Box 170, Beck Archives.

22. Ibid.

23. "Dr. Spivak Home Again," *The Sanatorium* 14 (July–September 1920): 26, JCRS Collection, Box 170, Beck Archives.

24. Dr. Philip Hillkowitz, "The President's Address," *The Sanatorium* 14 (July–September 1920): 26–27, JCRS Collection, Box 170, Beck Archives.

25. Dr. C. D. Spivak, "Sholom Aleichem," and "When the Editor Is Away," *The Sanatorium* 14 (October–December 1920): 34, JCRS Collection, Box 170, Beck Archives.

26. Dr. Chas. D. Spivak, "Health and Sanitation in the War-Stricken Countries," *The Sanatorium* 14 (October–December 1920): 35, 40, JCRS Collection, Box 170, Beck Archives.

27. "The Secretary's Trip to and from the Thirteenth Annual Meeting at Pittsburgh," *The Sanatorium* 11 (April–June 1917): 30, JCRS Collection, Box 170, Beck Archives.

28. C. D. Spivak, "The Annual Convention JCRS," JCRS Board of Trustees Minutes, April 25, 1921, JCRS Collection, Box 298, Beck Archives.

29. Ibid.

30. Ibid.

31. Isaac Rivkind, "The Last Days of Dr. Chayim Spivak," *The Sanatorium* 22 (October–December 1927); 12, JCRS Collection, Box 170, Beck Archives.

32. Dr. A. Levinson, "Dr. Chayim Spivak—Appreciation," *The Chicago Chronicle,* October 28, 1927.

33. Rivkind, "Last Days of Dr. Chayim Spivak," 13.

34. For a lively and informative look at *The Forward,* see the film *The Forward: From Immigrants to Americans,* directed by Marlene Booth (Los Angeles: Direct Cinema Limited, 1989).

35. *The Forward,* December 21, 1921.

36. Dr. Charles Spivak, "Dr. Spivak Proves That All the Commandments of the Torah Are Designed to Prolong Life," *The Forward,* April 16, 1922; "Washing Hands Is Not Only a Religious Observance," *The Forward,* June 11, 1922; "Don't Crawl into a Clean Bed with Dirty Feet," *The Forward,* June 25, 1922.

37. M. Sahud to Charles Spivak, March 20, 1922, JCRS Collection, Box 222, Beck Archives.

38. May Arno Schwatt, "The Violinist's Last Hour," *The Sanatorium* 5 (January–February 1911): 4–6, JCRS Collection, Box 170, Beck Archives.

39. May Schwatt to Charles Spivak, March 21, 1922, JCRS Collection, Box 222, Beck Archives.

40. Rosen and Miller to Charles Spivak, September 14, 1922, and Schwatt to Spivak, September 14, 1922, both in JCRS Collection, Box 222, Beck Archives.

41. Bellevue Hospital Record, September 26, 1922, JCRS Collection, Box 222, Beck Archives.

42. Dr. C. W. Thompson to Dr. C. D. Spivak, October 11, 18, and 22, 1922, JCRS Collection, Box 222, Beck Archives.

43. May Schwatt to Charles Spivak, October 3 and 30, 1922, JCRS Collection, Box 222, Beck Archives.

44. Dr. C. W. Thompson to Dr. C. D. Spivak, November 1, 9, and 15, 1922, JCRS Collection, Box 222, Beck Archives.

45. Interview with Adele Karsh conducted by Susan Goldman, May 29, 2005; interview with Adele Karsh and Eugene Spivak conducted by Jeanne Abrams, July 16, 2007.

46. Interview with Charlesa Wolfe Feinstein conducted by Jeanne Abrams, July 7, 2008.

47. H. Schwatt to Charles Spivak, November 7, 1925, JCRS Collection, Box 222, Beck Archives.

48. Dr. M. Sahud, "Dr. Spivak, the Saint," *The Sanatorium* (October–December 1927): 12, JCRS Collection, Box 170, Beck Archives.

49. National Conference of Jewish Social Service stationery, November 29, 1923, JCRS Collection, Box 222, Beck Archives.

50. "Federation Notes," undated, JCRS Collection, Box 222, Beck Archives.

51. C. D. Spivak, "The Federated Jewish Charities Movement in the United States," *The Sanatorium* 15 (October–December 1921): 41–45, JCRS Collection, Box 170, Beck Archives.

52. C. D. Spivak to Dr. B. Bogen, December 30, 1921, Spivak Collection, Beck Archives.

53. Dr. Boris Bogen to Dr. C. D. Spivak, January 4, 1922, Spivak Collection, Beck Archives.

54. *The Sanatorium* 16 (January–March 1922): 5, JCRS Collection, Box 170, Beck Archives.

55. Dr. C. D. Spivak, "The JCRS Launches a New Enterprise, a Home for All Ex-Patients Who Are Working," *The Sanatorium* 18 (October–December 1924): 91, JCRS Collection, Box 170, Beck Archives.

56. Quoted in *The Sanatorium* 22 (April–June 1927): 8, JCRS Collection, Box 170, Beck Archives.

57. Philip Hornbein to Dr. Spivak, March 12, 1927, JCRS Collection, Box 222, Beck Archives.

58. Philip Hillkowitz to Dr. Spivak, April 5, 1927, JCRS Collection, Box 222, Beck Archives.

59. Zion Commonwealth Land Certificate, September 24, 1917, and M. Esserman to Dr. C. D. Spivak, April 24, 1918, both in JCRS Collection, Box 222, Beck Archives.

60. S. J. Fox to Dr. C. D. Spivak, December 21, 1924, JCRS Collection, Box 222, Beck Archives.

61. *The Denver Jewish News,* November 28, 1918.

62. Rose Lurie to Charles Spivak, January 5, 1925, JCRS Collection, Box 222, Beck Archives.

63. Felix Warburg to Charles Spivak, August 12, 1925, JCRS Collection, Box 222, Beck Archives.

64. Victor Yarros, "Dr. Spivak's Early Days," *The Sanatorium* 22 (September–December 1927): 4, JCRS Collection, Box 170, Beck Archives.

65. Lulu Saul to Dr. D. Spivak, April 2, 1925, JCRS Collection, Box 222, Beck Archives.

66. C. D. Spivak, "A Bio-Ethnological Study of the Organized Medical Profession of the State of Colorado," *Colorado Medicine* 23 (1926).

67. *The Denver Jewish News,* November 19, 1919.

68. John Livingston, "Yiddishkeit along the Platte in the Jazz Age," *Rocky Mountain Jewish Historical Society Notes* 2–3 (January–April 1980): 8; Uchill, *Pioneers, Peddlers, and Tsadikim*, 231.

69. *The Denver Jewish News,* February 4, 1916.

70. *The Sanatorium* (October–December 1924): 104–105, JCRS Collection, Box 170, Beck Archives.

71. Uchill, *Pioneers, Peddlers, and Tsadikim*, 231.

72. Allen Breck, *A Centennial History of the Jews of Colorado* (Denver: Hirschfeld, 1960), 292.

73. Rivkind, "Last Days of Dr. Chayim Spivak," 14.

74. C. D. Spivak, "Longevity according to Hebrew Lore and Tradition," typescript manuscript, JCRS Collection, Box 222, Beck Archives.

CHAPTER 8: CONCLUSION: THE SPIVAK LEGACY

1. "Two Letters," *The Sanatorium* 22 (October–December 1927): 18, JCRS Collection, Box 170, Beck Archives, Special Collections, Penrose Library, University of Denver (hereafter Beck Archives).

2. *Rocky Mountain News* (Denver), October 18, 1927, clipping, Spivak Memorial Scrapbook, JCRS Collection, Box 222, Beck Archives.

3. "Memorial Meetings," *The Sanatorium* 22 (October–December 1929): 16, JCRS Collection, Box 170, Beck Archives.

4. *Rocky Mountain News* (Denver), October 18, 1927.

5. Ibid., November 17, 1927, clipping, Spivak Memorial Scrapbook, Box 222, JCRS Collection, Beck Archives.

6. For more information on Sewall, see Robert Shikes, *Rocky Mountain Medicine* (Boulder: Johnson Books, 1986), 127–128.

7. Dr. Henry Sewall, "Concerning Spivak," *Colorado Medicine* (December 1927), clipping, Spivak Memorial Scrapbook, JCRS Collection, Box 222, Beck Archives.

8. Cited in Isaac Rivkind, "The Last Days of Dr. Chayim Spivak," *The Sanatorium* 22 (October–December 1927): 12, JCRS Collection, Box 170, Beck Archives.

9. *The Intermountain Jewish News* (Denver), October 20, 1927, Spivak Memorial Scrapbook, JCRS Collection, Box 222, Beck Archives.

10. "Tribute to Dr. Spivak," *The Jewish Exponent* (Philadelphia), November 4, 1927, clipping, Spivak Memorial Scrapbook, JCRS Collection, Box 222, Beck Archives.

11. Ibid.

12. *Thirty Years of Saving Lives* (Denver: Jewish Consumptives' Relief Society, 1934), 23.

13. Spivak Memorial Scrapbook, JCRS Collection, Box 222, Beck Archives.

14. Ibid.

15. N. E. Mittenthal to the JCRS, October 17, 1927, JCRS Collection, Box 222, Beck Archives.

16. Philip Rossman to Mrs. C. D. Spivak and family, October 27, 1927, JCRS Collection, Box 222, Beck Archives.

17. Copy of Spivak Resolution, National Tuberculosis Association, January 16, 1928, JCRS Collection, Box 222, Beck Archives.

18. B'nai B'rith Memorial Resolution, JCRS Collection, Box 222, Beck Archives.

19. JCRS Board of Trustees Minutes, July 11, 1923, JCRS Collection, Box 298, Beck Archives.

20. Samuel Micon, "Dr. Chayim Spivak—Appreciation," *The Chicago Chronicle,* October 28, 1927, clipping, Spivak Memorial Scrapbook, JCRS Collection, Box 222, Beck Archives.

21. J. S. Shatz, "Editorial," *The Intermountain Jewish News* (Denver), November 10, 1927, clipping, Spivak Memorial Scrapbook, JCRS Collection, Box 222, Beck Archives.

22. For a detailed view of Goldberger's life and work, see Alan Kraut's fine biography, *Goldberger's War: The Life and Work of a Public Health Crusader* (New York: Hill and Wang, 2003).

23. Rivkind, "Last Days of Dr. Chayim Spivak," 12.

24. Rabbi William Friedman, "Spivak Obituary," *Jewish Monitor* (Fort Worth), October 28, 1927, Spivak Memorial Scrapbook, JCRS Collection, Box 222, Beck Archives.

25. Dr. A. Levinson, "Dr. Chayim Spivak—Appreciation," *The Chicago Chronicle,* October 28, 1927, clipping, Spivak Memorial Scrapbook, JCRS Collection, Box 222, Beck Archives.

26. Address by Rabbi William Friedman, 1923, Pisko File, National Jewish Hospital Collection, Beck Archives.

27. James Giese, "Tuberculosis and the Growth of Denver's Eastern European Jewish Community: The Accommodation of an Immigrant Group to a Medium-Sized Western City, 1900–1920," Ph.D. diss., University of Colorado, 1979, 130–134. Giese estimated, based on admittedly informal information, that as many as 60 percent of discharged NJH and JCRS patients remained in Denver, at least on a temporary basis.

28. Sheila M. Rothman, *Living in the Shadow of Death: Tuberculosis and the Social Experience of Illness in American History* (New York: Basic Books, 1994), 183.

29. Quoted in *Thirty Years of Saving Lives*, 23.

30. Alan M. Kraut, *Silent Travelers: Germs, Genes, and the "Immigrant Menace"* (New York: Basic Books, 1994), 190.

31. "Dr. Spivak's Talk," *The Sanatorium* 18 (October–December 1924): 102, JCRS Collection, Box 170, Beck Archives.

32. Alan M. Kraut, "No Matter How Poor and Small the Building: Health Care Institutions and the Jewish Immigrant Community," in Yvonne Yazbeck Haddad, Jane I. Smith, and John L. Esposito, eds., *Religion and Immigration: Christian, Jewish, and Muslim Experiences in the United States* (Walnut Creek, Calif.: Alta Mira, 2003), 130.

33. Alan M. Kraut, "Foreign Bodies: The Perennial Negotiation over Health and Culture in a Nation of Immigrants," *Journal of American Ethnic History* 23 (Winter 2004): 5.

34. Ibid., 5–7.

35. JCRS Annual Reports, 1905–1908, and Bureau of Social Research, *The Jewish Consumptives' Relief Society*, 1, both in JCRS Collection, Box 170, Beck Archives.

36. Katherine Ott, *Fevered Lives: Tuberculosis in American Culture since 1870* (Cambridge, Mass.: Harvard University Press, 1996), 149.

37. Nancy Tomes, *The Gospel of Germs: Men, Women, and the Microbe in American Life* (Cambridge, Mass.: Harvard University Press, 1998), 262.

38. Mark Caldwell, *The Last Crusade: The War on Consumption, 1862–1954* (New York: Atheneum, 1988).

39. Dr. Victor Yarros, "Dr. Spivak's Early Days," *The Sanatorium* 22 (October–December 1927): 3, JCRS Collection, Box 170, Beck Archives.

40. Dr. M. Sahud, "Spivak the Modern Saint," *The Sanatorium* 22 (October–December 1927): 12, JCRS Collection, Box 170, Beck Archives.

41. Dr. Charles Spivak, "The Genesis and Growth of the Jewish Consumptives' Relief Society," *The Sanatorium* 5 (July 1907): 190, JCRS Collection, Box 170, Beck Archives.

42. C. D. Spivak to Dr. J. B. Fish, August 31, 1909, JCRS Collection, Box 222, Beck Archives.

43. Agricultural Committee Minutes, April 25, 1925, 12, JCRS Collection, Box 168, Beck Archives.

44. David Rosner, *A Once Charitable Enterprise* (New York: Cambridge University Press, 1982), 42, chapter 3.

45. Philip Jacobs, *A Tuberculosis Directory* (New York: National Association for the Study and Prevention of Tuberculosis, 1911).

46. Thomas Galbreath, *T.B.: Playing the Lone Game Consumption* (New York: Journal of the Outdoor Life, 1915), 19.

47. Dr. Jay Sophro to Dr. Spivak, February 15, 1927, JCRS Collection, Box 222, Beck Archives.

48. Undated letter, Dr. Jay Sophro to Dr. Spivak, JCRS Collection, Box 222, Beck Archives.

49. Paula Hyman, "The Normalization of American Jewish History," *American Jewish History* 91 (2003): 355.

50. *Rocky Mountain News* (Denver), October 18, 1927.

51. For more on Einstein, see Walter Isaacson, *Einstein: His Life and Universe* (New York: Simon and Schuster, 2007).

Bibliography

PERIODICALS

The American Israelite (Cincinnati)
The Colorado Medical Journal
Colorado Medicine
The Denver Jewish News
Denver Medical News
The Denver Post
The Denver Republican
The Denver Times
The Forward (New York)
The Intermountain Jewish News (Denver)
The Jewish Exponent (Philadelphia)
The Jewish Messenger (New York)
Jewish Outlook (Denver)
Journal of the American Medical Association
Medical Libraries
Medical Life
The Philadelphia Inquirer

The Press (Philadelphia)
The Public Ledger (Philadelphia)
Rocky Mountain News
The Sanatorium (Denver) (JCRS)

MANUSCRIPT COLLECTIONS AND ORAL HISTORIES

B'nai B'rith of Denver Collection. Beck Archives, Special Collections, Penrose Library, University of Denver.

Feinstein, Charlesa Wolfe. Interview, July 7, 2008, conducted by Jeanne Abrams.

Frankel, Lee K., Papers. American Jewish Historical Society, New York, New York.

Glass, Ben, and Bessie Glass. Interview, October 22, 1978, conducted by Alby Segal. Beck Archives, Special Collections, Penrose Library, University of Denver.

Jewish Consumptives' Relief Society Collection. Beck Archives, Special Collections, Penrose Library, University of Denver. This entire collection is the most valuable resource on the life and work of Dr. Charles Spivak. The collection comprises over 300 record boxes, most containing relevant information of importance. Of particular value are Box 170, which includes JCRS publications and annual reports—most notably *The Sanatorium*—and Box 222, which contains the personal papers of Dr. Spivak.

Karsh, Adele. Interview, May 20, 2005, conducted by Susan Goldman.

National Jewish Hospital for Consumptives Collection. Beck Archives, Special Collections, Penrose Library, University of Denver.

Spivak, Dr. Charles David, Papers. Beck Archives, Special Collections, Penrose Library, University of Denver.

Spivak, Eugene, and Adele Strauss Karsh. Interview, July 16, 2007, conducted by Jeanne Abrams.

Strauss, Deena Spivak. Interview, March 13, 1982, conducted by Jeanne Abrams. #90, Oral History Collection, Beck Archives, Special Collections, Penrose Library, University of Denver.

University of Denver Bulletins, 1903–1913. Special Collections, Penrose Library, University of Denver.

PUBLISHED PRIMARY SOURCES

Axtell, E. R. "Tent Life for Consumptives." *The Colorado Climatologist* 1 (May 1895): 159–161.

Ball, Edward L., diary transcriber. *The Life of Michael Valentine Ball, 1868–1945.* Warren, Pa.: self-published, 2003.

Bogen, Boris. *Born a Jew.* New York: Macmillan, 1930.

———. *Jewish Philanthropy.* New York: Macmillan, 1917.

Bonney, Sherman. "What Consumptives Should Come to Colorado?" *Denver Medical Times* 28 (October 1908): 144–147.

Denison, Charles. "How Does Climate Influence Tuberculosis?" *Denver Medical Times* 28 (1908): 141–144.

Denver Chamber of Commerce. *Fourth Annual Report.* Denver: Chamber of Commerce, 1887.

Fishberg, Maurice. "Tuberculosis among the Jews." *American Medicine* 2 (1901): 695–699.

Freeman, Moses. *Fuftzig Yohr Geshikhte fun Yidishn Leben in Filadelfia*, Vol. I. Philadelphia: Posy-Shoulson, 1929.

Galbreath, Thomas. *Chasing the Cure in Colorado.* Denver: self-published, 1907.

———. *T.B.: Playing the Lone Game Consumption.* New York: Journal of the Outdoor Life, 1915.

Jacobs, Philip. *A Tuberculosis Directory.* New York: National Association for the Study and Prevention of Tuberculosis, 1911.

Magruder, A. J. "Physicians in Colorado for Tuberculosis." *Denver Medical Times* 28 (October 1908): 152–153.

Sewall, Dr. Henry. "Concerning Spivak." *Colorado Medicine* (December 1927): 378.

Spivak, Dr. Charles. "A Bio-Ethnological Study of the Organized Medical Profession of the State of Colorado." *Colorado Medicine* 23 (1926): 188–194.

———. "The Medical Libraries of the United States." *Medical Libraries Supplement* (January 1899): 1.

———. "Medical Reprints." *Journal of the American Medical Association* 39 (1902: 1018.

———. "Rest—A Neglected Factor in the Treatment of Gastro-Intestinal Disorder." *Journal of the American Medical Association* 21 (July 30, 1898): 216.

———. "The Union Catalogue of Medical Books, and Some of the Private Medical Libraries in the City of Denver," *The Colorado Medical Journal* 3 (1897): 214.

Spivakovsky, Chaim. "On the Way in an American Factory." *Rocky Mountain Jewish Historical Notes* 16 (Summer-Fall 2001): 1–8.

Teller, Jacob Chester. *Report on the Problem of Combined Poverty and Tuberculosis among Jews in Denver, Colorado.* New York: National Conference of Jewish Charities, 1916.

Trudeau, Edward. *An Autobiography.* New York: Doubleday, Page, 1916.

Tuberculosis in Denver. Denver: Health Committee of the City Club of Denver, 1925.

Weinstein, Gregory. *The Ardent Eighties and After; Reminiscences of a Busy Life.* New York: International Press, 1947.

Woods, Luther H. "Seeking Health in Colorado." *Denver Medical Times* 18 (May 1899): 535–537.

SECONDARY SOURCES

Abel, Emily K. "Medicine and Morality: The Health Care Program of the New York Charity Organization Society." *Social Service Review* 4 (December 1997): 634–651.

Abrams, Jeanne. *Blazing the Tuberculosis Trail.* Denver: Colorado Historical Society, 1990.

———. "Chasing the Cure: A History of the Jewish Consumptives' Relief Society of Denver." Ph.D. diss., University of Colorado at Boulder, 1984.

———. *Jewish Women Pioneering the Frontier Trail: A History in the American West.* New York: New York University Press, 2006.

Anfenger, Milton. *The Birth of a Hospital: The Story of the Birth of the National Jewish Hospital in Denver.* Denver: National Jewish Hospital, 1943.

Barnes, David. *The Making of a Disease: Tuberculosis in Nineteenth Century France.* Berkeley: University of California Press, 1995.

Barth, Gunther. *Instant Cities: Urbanization and the Rise of San Francisco and Denver.* New York: Oxford University Press, 1975.

Bates, Barbara. *Bargaining for Life: A Social History of Tuberculosis, 1876–1938.* Philadelphia: University of Pennsylvania Press, 1992.

Berger, David, ed. *The Legacy of Jewish Migration: 1881 and Its Impact.* New York: Brooklyn College Press, 1983.

Boggs, Alice. "The History and Development of the Tuberculosis Assistance Program in Colorado." M.A. thesis, University of Denver, 1943.

Boonin, Harry. *The Jewish Quarter of Philadelphia.* Philadelphia: Jewish Walking Tours of Philadelphia, 1999.

Brandes, Joseph. *Immigrants to Freedom: Jewish Communities in Rural New Jersey since 1882.* Philadelphia: University of Pennsylvania Press, 1971.

Breck, Allen. *A Centennial History of the Jews of Colorado.* Denver: Hirschfeld, 1960.

Bremner, Robert. *Children and Youth in America: A Documentary History*, Vol. II: *1866–1923.* Cambridge, Mass.: Harvard University Press, 1971 [1903].

Bridge, Daniel Ethan. "The Rise and Development of the Jewish Hospital in America." Rabbinic Ordination thesis, Hebrew Union College, 1985.

Buenker, John D., John C. Burnham, and Robert M. Cruden, eds. *Progressivism.* Cambridge, Mass.: Harvard University Press, 1977.

Cahan, Abraham. *The Education of Abraham Cahan.* Philadelphia: Jewish Publication Society of America, 1969.

Caldwell, Mark. *The Last Crusade: The War on Consumption, 1862–1954.* New York: Atheneum, 1988.

Cassedy, Steven. *To the Other Shore: The Russian Jewish Intellectuals Who Came to America.* Princeton, N.J.: Princeton University Press, 1997.

Cohen, Naomi. *Encounter with Emancipation.* Philadelphia: Jewish Publication Society, 1984.

———. *Not Free to Desist.* Philadelphia: Jewish Publication Society, 1972.

Crevecouer, Hector St. John. *Letters from an American Farmer.* New York: E. P. Dutton, 1912.

Daniel, Thomas M. *Captain of Death: The Story of Tuberculosis.* Rochester, N.Y.: University of Rochester Press, 1999.

Daniels, Roger. *Coming to America: A History of Immigration and Ethnicity in American Life.* New York: Harper Perennial, 1991.

Diner, Hasia R. *Hungering for America: Italian, Irish, and Jewish Foodways in the Age of Migration.* Cambridge, Mass.: Harvard University Press, 2001.

Dormandy, Thomas. *The White Death, a History of Tuberculosis.* New York: New York University Press, 2000.

Drolit, Godias J. *Tuberculosis Hospitalization.* New York: New York Tuberculosis and Health Association, 1926.

Dubois, Renee, and Jean Dubois. *The White Plague: Man and Society.* Boston: Little, Brown, 1952.

Feldberg, Georgina. *Disease and Class: Tuberculosis and the Shaping of Modern North American Society.* New Brunswick, N.J.: Rutgers University Press, 1995.

Filene, David. "An Obituary for the 'Progressive Movement.'" *American Quarterly* 22 (Spring 1970): 20–34.

Fitzharris, Mary Ann, and Jeanne Abrams. *A Place to Heal: A History of National Jewish Medical and Research Center.* Boulder: Johnson, 1998.

Flexner, Abraham. *Medical Education in the United States and Canada: A Report to the Carnegie Foundation for the Advancement of Teaching.* Bulletin 4. New York: Carnegie Foundation, reprint, 1972 [1910].

Frankel, Jonathan. *Prophesy and Politics.* New York: Cambridge University Press, 1981.

Friedman, Murray, ed. *Jewish Life in Philadelphia.* Philadelphia: Jewish Publication Society, 1983.

Gandy, Matthew. "Life without Germs: Contested Episodes in the History of Tuberculosis." In Matthew Gandy and Alimuddin Zumla, *The Return of the White Plague: Global Poverty and the "New" Tuberculosis.* New York: Verso, 2003, 15–38.

Geffen, Joel S. "Whither: To Palestine or to America in the Pages of the Russian Hebrew Press *Ha-Melitz* and *Ha-Yom* (1880–1890)." *American Jewish Historical Quarterly* 59 (December 1969): 179–200.

Giese, James. "Tuberculosis and the Growth of Denver's Eastern European Jewish Community: The Accommodation of an Immigrant Group to a Medium-Sized Western City, 1900–1920." Ph.D. diss., University of Colorado, 1979.

Harkavy, Alexander. "Chapters from My Life." *American Jewish Archive* 17 (April 1981): 33–37.

Harper, Fred. *The Story of Tuberculosis and the Evangelical Lutheran Sanitarium.* Denver: Lutheran Hospital, 1980.

Hart, Mitchell Bryan. *The Healthy Jew: The Symbiosis of Judaism and Modern Medicine.* New York: Cambridge University Press, 2007.

The Heart of the Rockies. Denver: Denver & Rio Grande Railroad, 1880.

Herscher, Uri D. *Jewish Agricultural Utopias in America.* Detroit: Wayne State University Press, 1981.

Hertzberg, Arthur. *The Jews in America.* New York: Simon and Schuster, 1989.

Hillkowitz, Philip. "Charles David Spivak, 1861–1927." *The American Review of Tuberculosis* 16 (December 1927): 763–765.

Hornbein, Marjorie. "Dr. Charles Spivak of Denver: Physician, Social Worker, Yiddish Author." *Western States Jewish Historical Quarterly* 11 (April 1977): 193–204.

———. "Frances Jacobs: Denver's Mother of Charities." *Western States Jewish Historical Quarterly* 14 (January 1983): 131–145.

Hyman, Paula. "The Normalization of American Jewish History." *American Jewish History* 91 (2003): 353–359.

Isaacson, Walter. *Einstein: His Life and Universe.* New York: Simon and Schuster, 2007.

Jones, Billy. *Health Seekers in the Southwest, 1817–1900.* Norman: University of Oklahoma Press, 1967.

Karp, Abraham. *Golden Door to America: The Jewish Immigrant Experience.* New York: Viking, 1976.

Kerber, Linda. "Separate Spheres, Female Worlds, Woman's Place: The Rhetoric of Women's History." *The Journal of American History* 75 (June 1988): 9–39.

Knopf, S. Adoldphus. *Tuberculosis as a Disease of the Masses and How to Combat It.* New York: M. Firestack, 1901.

Kobrin, Leon. *A Lithuanian Village.* New York: Bernard G. Richards, 1927.

———. *Mayne Fuftsik Yor in Amerike.* Buenos Aires: Yidbukh bay der Gezelshaft far Yidish-Veltlekhe Shuln in Argentine, 1955.

Kraut, Alan M. "Foreign Bodies: The Perennial Negotiation over Health and Culture in a Nation of Immigrants." *Journal of American Ethnic History* 23 (Winter 2004): 3–22.

———. *Goldberger's War: The Life and Work of a Public Health Crusader.* New York: Hill and Wang, 2003.

———. "No Matter How Poor and Small the Building: Health Care Institutions and the Jewish Immigrant Community." In Yvonne Yazbeck Haddad, Jane I. Smith, and John L. Esposito, eds., *Religion and Immigration: Christian, Jewish, and Muslim Experiences in the United States.* Walnut Creek, Calif.: Alta Mira, 2003, 129–158.

———. *Silent Travelers: Germs, Genes, and the "Immigrant Menace."* New York: Basic Books, 1994.

Leavitt, Judith Walzer, and Ronald L. Numbers, eds. *Sickness and Health in America: Readings in the History of Medicine and Public Health*, 3rd ed. Madison: University of Wisconsin Press, 1997.

Levin, Nora. *While Messiah Tarried: The Jewish Socialist Movements, 1871–1917.* New York: Schocken Books, 1977.

Lindenthal, Jacob. "Abi Gezunt: Health and the Eastern European Jewish Immigrant." *American Jewish History* 70 (June 1981): 420–441.

Livingston, John. "Yiddishkeit along the Platte in the Jazz Age." *Rocky Mountain Jewish Historical Notes* 2–3 (January-April 1980): 7–11.

Ludemerer, Kenneth M. *A Time to Heal: American Medical Education from the Turn of the Century to the Era of Managed Care.* New York: Oxford University Press, 1999.

McKay, Douglas R. *Asylum of the Gilded Pill.* Denver: Colorado Historical Society, 1983.

———. "A History of the Nordrach Ranch: Colorado's First Sanatorium of the Open Air." *The Colorado Magazine* 56 (Summer-Fall 1979): 179–195.

Mead, Rebecca. *How the Vote Was Won.* New York: New York University Press, 2004.

Memoirs of Frances Jacobs. Denver: Charity Organization Society, 1892.

Mendelsohn, Ezra. *Class Struggle in the Pale: The Formative Years of the Jewish Worker's Movement in Tsarist Russia.* London: Cambridge University Press, 1970.

———. "The Russian Roots of the American Jewish Labor Movement." *YIVO Annual of Jewish Social Science* 16 (1976): 150–177.

Menes, Abraham. "The Am Olam Movement." *YIVO Annual of Jewish Social Science* 4 (1949): 9–33.

Michels, Tony. *A Fire in Their Hearts: Yiddish Socialists in New York.* Cambridge, Mass.: Harvard University Press, 2005.

Mitman, Gregg. "Geographies of Hope: Mining the Frontiers of Health in Denver and Beyond, 1870–1965." *Osiris* 19 (2004): 93–111.

Nathans, Benjamin. *Beyond the Pale: The Jewish Encounter with Late Imperial Russia.* Berkeley: University of California Press, 2002.

———. "The Jews." In Dominic Lieven, ed., *The Cambridge History of Russia,* Vol. II, *Imperial Russia, 1689–1917.* New York: Cambridge University Press, 2006, 184–202.

Ogren, Christine A. "A Large Measure of Self-Control and Personal Power: Women Students at State Normal Schools during the Late-Nineteenth and Early-Twentieth Century." *Women's Studies Quarterly* 18 (Fall-Winter 2000): 211–227.

Ott, Katherine. *Fevered Lives: Tuberculosis in American Culture since 1870.* Cambridge, Mass.: Harvard University Press, 1996.

Reversby, Susan, and David Rosner. *Health Care in America.* Philadelphia: Temple University Press, 1979.

Rischin, Moses, and John Livingston, eds. *Jews of the American West.* Detroit: Wayne State University Press, 1991.

Rogow, Faith. *Gone to Another Meeting: The National Council of Jewish Women, 1890–1993.* Tuscaloosa: University of Alabama Press, 1993.

Rosenberg. Charles. *The Care of Strangers: The Rise of America's Hospital System.* New York: Basic Books, 1987.

Rosner, David. *A Once Charitable Enterprise.* New York: Cambridge University Press, 1982.

Rothman, Sheila M. *Living in the Shadow of Death: Tuberculosis and the Social Experience of Illness in American History.* New York: Basic Books, 1994.

Ryan, Frank. *The Forgotten Plague: How the Battle against Tuberculosis Was Won—and Lost.* Boston: Little, Brown, 1993.

Sarna, Jonathan. *American Judaism.* New Haven: Yale University Press, 2004.

Shikes, Robert. *Rocky Mountain Medicine.* Boulder: Johnson, 1986.

Smith, Henry Nash. *Virgin Land, the American West as Symbol and Myth.* New York: Vintage Books, 1950.

Sombart, Werner. *Why Is There No Socialism in the United States.* White Plains, N.Y.: International Arts and Science Press, 1976 [1906].

Sorin, Gerald. *The Prophetic Minority: American Jewish Immigrant Radicals, 1880–1920.* Bloomington: Indiana University Press, 1985.

———. "Review of *A Fire in Their Hearts.*" *American Jewish History* 92 (September 2006): 383–386.

Szasz, Ferenc Morton. *Religion in the Modern American West.* Tucson: University of Arizona Press, 2000.

Tandy, Francis. "The Colorado Medical Library Association." *Medical Libraries* 1 (May 1898): 27.

Teller, Michael. *The Tuberculosis Movement: A Public Health Campaign in the Progressive Era.* New York: Greenwood, 1988.

Thirty Years of Saving Lives. Denver: Jewish Consumptives' Relief Society, 1934.

Tomes, Nancy. *The Gospel of Germs: Men, Women, and the Microbe in American Life.* Cambridge, Mass.: Harvard University Press, 1998.

Uchill, Ida. *Pioneers, Peddlers, and Tsadikim.* Denver: Sage, 1959.

Varney, George J. "History of Lisbon, Maine." In *Gazetteer of the State of Maine.* Boston: B. B. Russell, 1886, 333–336.

Wiernik, Peter. *History of the Jews in America.* New York: Jewish Press Publishing, 1912.

Wirth-Nesher, Hana. *Call It English: The Language of Jewish American Literature.* Princeton, N.J.: Princeton University Press, 2006.

Zelinger, Michael. *West Side Story Relived.* Denver: Wandel, 1987.

Index

Page numbers in italics indicate illustrations.